BEYOND CHEMISTRY

Hormones, Healing & Human Connection in the Age of Disconnection

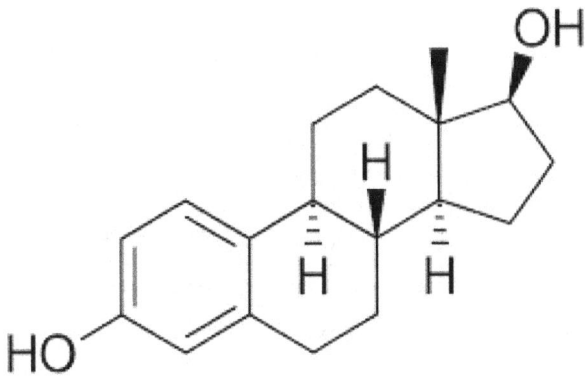

By: Dr. Deilen Michelle Villegas, Ph.D.

For permissions, contact publisher:
The Shamanic Goddess, LLC
Charlotte, North Carolina, United States
www.DrDeilenMVillegas.com
Dr.Deilen.Villegas@gmail.com

This book is intended for educational and informational purposes only. It is not a substitute for professional medical advice, diagnosis, or treatment. Always seek the guidance of your physician or qualified health provider with any questions you may have regarding a medical condition. The author disclaims any liability arising directly or indirectly from the use of this book.

Book Title: Beyond Chemistry: Hormones, Healing & Human Connection in the Age of Disconnection
Author: Dr. Deilen Michelle Villegas, Ph.D.
Publisher: The Shamanic Goddess, LLC
Cover and Interior Design: The Shamanic Goddess, LLC

ISBN: 978-1-969550-01-0
First Edition: 2026
Printed in the United States of America

About The Author

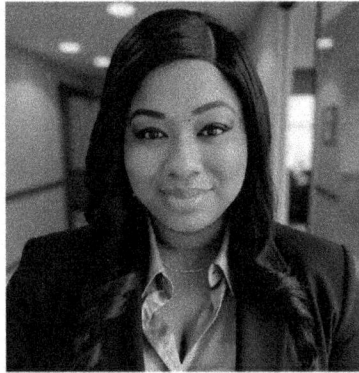

Dr. Deilen Michelle Villegas, Ph.D., is a Board-Certified Holistic Health Practitioner, Clinical Mental Health Counselor, Trauma Specialist, and Certified Sexologist. With over 18 years of combined clinical and holistic experience, she stands at the intersection of science, spirituality, and integrative healing.

As the visionary Founder and CEO of The Shamanic Goddess, LLC, Dr. Villegas has dedicated her life to empowering individuals and communities, especially those historically marginalized, to reclaim their vitality, emotional resilience, and sacred embodiment. Her diverse academic background includes a Ph.D. in Metaphysical Sciences and Natural Health, a Ph.D. in Organizational Leadership, an M.A. in Clinical Mental Health Counseling, and an M.S. in Complementary & Integrative Medicine.

Dr. Villegas is known for her unapologetic approach to healing, her commitment to cultural competence, and her ability to fuse ancient wisdom with modern science. Through her books, programs, and client work, she invites others to explore the full spectrum of what it means to be human—raw, radiant, complex, and connected.

She is also a devoted mother, advocate, and spiritual practitioner who believes that healing is both a personal revolution and a collective responsibility.

Connect with Dr. Deilen:

Website: www.drdeilenmvillegas.com
Instagram: @author_dr_deilen_m_villegas

Other titles by the author:

- *Reclaiming the Unspoken: The Journey Through Trauma, Truth & Transformation*

- *Rewired for Resilience: The Neurosomatic Path to Healing, Embodiment, and Transformation*

- *Rooted In Wisdom: Holistic Herbal Medicine For The Healing Communities*

- *Awakened Science: Where Quantum Physics Meets the Divine*

- *Sacred Flesh: The Science, Spirit, and Power of Intimacy*

- *She Who Became: The Verses of a Wild Woman*

- *Encoded In The Stars: The Science of Destiny and the Blueprint of the Soul*

Dedication

To the ones who feel too much,
love too deeply,
and dream of a world more connected than the one we've
inherited.

To every woman, man, and soul in between
who has questioned their worth, their wiring, or their
wellness
in a world that forgot the sacredness of the human experience.

To the healers reclaiming their medicine,
the seekers redefining science,
and the visionaries daring to bridge biology with the divine.

May this work remind you:
You are not broken.
You are becoming.
You are beyond chemistry.

With deepest gratitude,
I dedicate this book to my ancestors,
whose whispers echo through my work,
and to my children,
whose futures I write into every page.

— *Dr. Deilen Michelle Villegas*

Table Of Contents

About The Author

Dedication

Preface: A Personal Invitation to Reconnection

Introduction: Why This Book, Why Now?

Chapter 1: The Polarity of Human Behavior

Chapter 2: Relationships & Hormonal Interplay

Chapter 3: Estrogen, Progesterone & Testosterone: Foundations & Imbalances

Chapter 4: Postpartum Depression & Hormonal Shifts

Chapter 5: Medication & Post-SSRI Sexual Dysfunction

Chapter 6: Infertility & Hidden Root Causes

Chapter 7: Modern Day Infertility—Lifestyle Therapy as Medicine

Chapter 8: Menopause & Mortality – The Unspoken Transition

Chapter 9: Profiling Hypo-Function in Males

Chapter 10: Male Pattern Hair Loss & What It Reveals

Chapter 11: The Crisis of Traditional Masculinity

Chapter 12: Prostate Health, Erectile Function, & True Libido

Chapter 13: Libido, Emotional Intimacy & Relational Polarity Across Genders

Chapter 14: Integrating Hormone Harmony, Healing, and Soul-Aligned Relationships

Chapter 15: Rebalancing Through Lifestyle Medicine

Chapter 16: The Sacred Return to Self-Integrating Masculine & Feminine

Acknowledgements

Appendices

- Comprehensive Glossary of Terms
- Assessments & Checklist
- Worksheets
- Protocols and Daily Support Plans
- Libido & Hormone Tracking Tools
- Healing Roadmap: Reclaiming Hormonal Balance, Connection, and Wholeness

Preface: A Personal Invitation To Reconnection

I wrote this book for the seekers, the ones who've been told their pain is "normal," their pleasure isn't a priority, and their hormones are just "crazy." I wrote it for the women craving clarity, the men silencing their fatigue, and the couples losing their connection to stress and shame. I wrote it as a practitioner, a counselor, a sexologist, and as a woman who has lived the disconnection and fought her way back to wholeness.

This book is not just about hormones. It is about chemistry —the electric spark between biology and behavior, emotion and energy, connection and chaos. It's about how trauma shapes our endocrine system, how chronic stress mutates into disease, and how relationships can regulate or rupture our nervous systems. It's about the narratives we inherit, the cultural silence around pleasure and fatigue, and the invisible weight that so many carry in their minds, hearts, and reproductive systems.

It's also about reclamation. About choosing to remember that our bodies are sacred, intelligent, and worthy of care. That pleasure is not a luxury but a language—a way the body speaks when it feels safe, seen, and sovereign. That hormonal health is not isolated from mental health, spiritual alignment, or sexual freedom.

"Beyond Chemistry" is an unapologetic, research-backed, spiritually infused call to come home to yourself. It blends the science of hormonal healing with the soul of human connection. Whether you're a clinician, a client, a curious soul, or a partner navigating intimacy, you belong here. If you've ever felt dismissed, misdiagnosed, or disconnected from your body's wisdom, this book is your mirror and your medicine.

Inside these pages, we explore the clinical and the cosmic— from neurotransmitters to neurotransmissions of spirit. We will sit with the complexity of hormonal shifts, the grief that sometimes accompanies change, and the glory that returns when we learn to listen. We'll examine cultural myths, break taboos, and build bridges between science and spirituality, the masculine and the feminine, the brain and the body.

May this book open your eyes, nourish your truth, and call you back into the rhythm of your own body, your own joy, and your own sacred connections. May it be the reminder you didn't know you needed—that you are not broken, you are becoming.

With reverence and purpose,

—**Dr. Deilen Michelle Villegas, Ph.D.**

INTRODUCTION

Why This Book, Why Now?

We are living in an era of overexposure and underconnection. Hormonal imbalances are on the rise. Infertility is increasing. Sexual dysfunction is becoming normalized, even expected. Meanwhile, social media glorifies youth and perfection, leaving many adults secretly struggling with shame, fatigue, and silent disconnection.

This is not just a medical crisis—it is a relational and spiritual one.

As a Board-Certified Holistic Health Practitioner, Clinical Mental Health Counselor, and Certified Sexologist, I've sat with hundreds of clients who whisper the same questions:

"Why don't I feel like myself anymore?" "Where did my desire go?" "Why can't we connect like we used to?" "Is this just aging, or is something wrong with me?"

The truth is: Our bodies are talking. And they've been trying to get our attention for years.

This book bridges the gaps between clinical insight, holistic care, and soul-aligned living. Each chapter blends anatomy, neuroscience, endocrinology, trauma research, and energetic healing practices into a full-spectrum lens for understanding the interconnectedness of hormones, health, sexuality, and human behavior.

You'll find:

- Peer-reviewed studies and functional medicine insights
- Case studies from real-life clinical practice
- Cultural reflections on masculinity, femininity, fertility,

and censorship
- Tools for regulation, rejuvenation, and relational intimacy

This book is not about perfection. It's about *permission*, to heal, to change, to explore, to feel, and to thrive.

You are not broken. You are becoming.

Let's begin the journey *beyond chemistry*—and back into connection.

CHAPTER 1

The Polarity of Human Behavior

Understanding the Spectrum

Human behavior is not binary. It exists on a fluid spectrum, shaped by a complex interplay of hormones, neurobiology, early conditioning, cultural expectation, and lived experience. In clinical settings, we often encounter clients struggling to reconcile the natural polarity of their behavior—masculine and feminine energies, assertiveness and receptivity, logic and emotion. This chapter navigates the biological, psychological, and social roots of these polarities and their importance in the healing process.

Polarity, in this context, refers to the dynamic tension between opposing but complementary forces within human identity. It is neither about gender nor sexual orientation—it is about energetic tendencies, neural dominance, and hormone-driven behavioral expression. Masculine and feminine polarities exist in all bodies, regardless of sex, and they influence everything from decision-making to intimacy and stress responses. The healthy expression of polarity supports resilience, identity integration, and relational depth.

We live in a culture that often pathologizes polarity—labeling assertiveness as aggression, sensitivity as weakness, and emotionality as instability. Yet these polarities are essential to human wholeness. When we suppress one side of the spectrum, we create internal dissonance, which can manifest as anxiety, depression, burnout, or relational disconnection. In contrast, when we embrace our full range of energies and expressions, we step into greater authenticity, fluidity, and self-compassion.

Masculine energy, classically associated with focus, direction, and structure, is governed in part by testosterone and dopamine-driven pathways. Feminine energy, associated with intuition, creativity, and nurturing, is supported by estrogen, oxytocin, and the parasympathetic nervous system. Both energies serve vital biological and psychological roles, and both can be cultivated consciously, regardless of one's assigned sex at birth.

Therapeutically, the recognition and integration of polarity becomes a powerful tool. Clients who have disowned their assertiveness due to trauma or socialization may find empowerment by reclaiming their inner fire. Others who've over-identified with performance, productivity, or hyper-independence may discover healing in surrendering to rest, receptivity, and emotional expression.

In relationships, polarity creates magnetic charge—the dance between giver and receiver, structure and flow. When partners become energetically neutralized, intimacy may dwindle, and communication may suffer. Learning to embody and respect each partner's unique energetic rhythm can restore passion, safety, and mutual growth.

From a clinical perspective, unresolved polarity conflicts often mirror deeper attachment wounds, familial modeling, and cultural programming. A woman raised to perform in masculine-coded environments may struggle with vulnerability. A man socialized to suppress his emotions may feel lost in moments requiring tenderness or attunement. Gender expansive and nonbinary individuals, too, navigate the terrain of polarity with profound courage and fluidity, often holding the wisdom of integration within their lived experience.

As practitioners, our role is to hold space for clients to explore these inner tensions—not to force alignment with outdated roles or rigid expectations, but to support self-discovery and embodied balance. We are guiding people back to their nature, not to a norm.

Key Reflections:

- Where have I over-identified with one aspect of polarity?
- What parts of me feel suppressed or unsafe to express?
- How do my hormonal cycles affect my emotional and energetic polarity?
- Where in my life do I need more structure? Where do I need more flow?

Clinical Application: Use polarity mapping as a therapeutic tool. Chart behaviors, language patterns, and somatic tendencies across masculine/feminine spectra. Support clients in identifying how stress, trauma, or hormone shifts may influence their expression of polarity. Teach clients to access the polarity they most need in the moment—using breathwork, movement, or cognitive reframing.

"The goal of therapy is not to neutralize polarity, but to integrate it." — Dr. Deilen Michelle Villegas

Neuroscience and Hormonal Foundations of Polarity

Biologically, sex hormones such as testosterone, estrogen, and progesterone play pivotal roles in shaping how we perceive the world and respond to stimuli. Testosterone is often associated with assertiveness, spatial orientation, risk-taking, and focused attention. Estrogen, on the other hand, enhances verbal fluency, emotional nuance, social bonding, and sensory receptivity. Progesterone, frequently overlooked in public discourse, plays a calming role—supporting sleep, mood stabilization, and resilience to stress by modulating GABA receptors (Bäckström et al., 2011).

Importantly, these hormones exist in all bodies—just in different ratios—and they fluctuate based on life stage, circadian rhythms, menstrual or hormonal cycles, stress exposure, and even interpersonal interactions. This means that polarity is not a fixed trait but a dynamic expression shaped by internal and external environments. For example, cortisol, the stress hormone, can suppress both testosterone and estrogen production, leading to emotional dysregulation and decreased libido—clear evidence that modern stressors can blur our internal polarity expression (Sapolsky, 2004).

Recent studies have emphasized that the effects of sex hormones are not exclusive to one gender. Men produce estrogen, which is critical for brain development, sperm maturation, and modulating aggression. Women produce testosterone, which supports libido, motivation, and muscle repair. The synergy of these hormones—and the balance between them—is what truly governs behavior, not their mere presence (Bangasser & Cuarenta, 2021).

From a neuroanatomical standpoint, functional MRI studies show distinct but complementary patterns in brain connectivity influenced by hormonal profiles. Women tend to exhibit more **cross-hemispheric connectivity**, linking the left (logical) and right (intuitive) hemispheres. This supports multitasking, emotional integration, and social cognition. Men more often display **intra-hemispheric dominance**, supporting systemized thinking, task-specific focus, and compartmentalization (Ingalhalikar et al., 2014). These differences are not rigid and should not be interpreted as superior or inferior—rather, they represent natural variations in processing style and behavioral polarity.

Moreover, these neurological patterns are **neuroplastic**— meaning they can shift over time in response to trauma, healing, hormonal interventions, and somatic practices. A person recovering from emotional suppression may show increased connectivity in the limbic system, enhancing emotional awareness. Similarly, meditation and breathwork have been shown to increase prefrontal-limbic integration, improving both impulse control and emotional regulation (Tang, Hölzel, & Posner, 2015).

For example, clients with early childhood trauma may experience dysregulated HPA axis activity (hypothalamic-pituitary-adrenal), resulting in chronic overactivation of survival states—fight, flight, or freeze. This dysregulation may diminish testosterone levels in men or progesterone levels in women, skewing their behavioral polarities toward anxiety, emotional blunting, or burnout. Trauma-focused interventions, such as somatic experiencing or neurofeedback, can help recalibrate these systems and restore access to a more integrated range of polarity.

From a clinical lens, understanding the **neuroendocrine basis of polarity** allows us to normalize diverse behaviors and responses, especially during hormonal transitions such as puberty, postpartum, perimenopause, and andropause. Rather than viewing mood shifts or libido changes as dysfunctions, we begin to understand them as reflections of the body's attempt to rebalance and protect itself.

Key Takeaway:
Polarity is not a binary dictated by gender; it is a biologically intelligent dance between hormones and neurons, spirit and soma. When we learn to decode our internal chemistry, we reclaim the ability to live and love from an empowered place of integration rather than fragmentation.

Polarity in Relationships and Identity

From romantic dynamics to parenting styles, polarity profoundly influences our relational blueprints. These energetic patterns are not simply personality quirks—they are deeply rooted expressions of our hormonal environment, nervous system state, early attachment conditioning, and cultural learning. The interplay of masculine and feminine energies is evident in how couples navigate intimacy, conflict, boundaries, and support.

When one partner consistently over-functions in one polarity—such as always leading, providing, initiating, or emotionally containing—the relational dynamic can become rigid or lopsided. Over time, this dynamic may lead to **resentment, emotional burnout, or sexual disconnection.** The tension arises not because one polarity is "wrong," but because sustainable relationships require *fluidity*—a mutual attunement to shifting needs, roles, and emotional capacities.

Healthy polarity in relationships is not about conforming to gender norms but rather cultivating complementary energies that allow each person to feel **seen, supported, and self-expressed.** Feminine polarity (regardless of gender) brings in intuition, empathy, sensual presence, and emotional resonance. Masculine polarity contributes direction, protection, containment, and clarity. In conscious relationships, these energies dance—not dominate.

Case Study: Derek

Derek, a 38-year-old Black male client, presented with symptoms of emotional withdrawal, fatigue, and relationship avoidance. He expressed feeling "used up" at work and "emotionally numb" at home. Raised in a home where vulnerability was punished and stoicism praised, Derek had internalized the belief that his value lay in his productivity and emotional restraint.

In therapy, it became clear that Derek had unconsciously suppressed his "feminine" polarity—nurturance, emotional expression, and receptivity—believing these traits to be signs of weakness or danger. While he consistently provided for his family and met logistical needs, his partners often described him as emotionally unavailable or disengaged. This disconnect contributed to mounting relational tension, intimacy avoidance, and chronic insomnia.

Using an integrative approach, we introduced somatic tracking, guided breathwork, and polarity mapping. Derek began to recognize when his nervous system braced against softness—especially during moments of potential emotional vulnerability. Through safe, structured exercises (including mirroring, inner child dialogues, and expressive journaling), he began reawakening a fuller range of emotional intelligence.

Over time, Derek not only initiated deeper conversations with his partner but also expressed affection more freely, took creative risks (such as returning to music), and learned to receive without shame. His libido improved. His sleep deepened. His relational presence transformed.

> "When I stopped trying to be the strong one all the time, I realized how tired I really was—and how good it felt to be held, too." — Derek, client reflection

This reintegration of polarity wasn't just relational—it was biological. As Derek's vagus nerve regulation improved through breath and somatic work, his symptoms of anxiety and hypervigilance decreased. His testosterone levels stabilized. He stopped grinding his teeth at night. These shifts reflect the deep truth: **when we live in energetic congruence, the body begins to heal.**

Identity and the Internal Polarity Conflict

Polarity is not just a dynamic between people—it's a dialogue within the self.

Many individuals, particularly those socialized in high-achievement, hyper-masculinized, or survival-based environments, learn to **disown one side of their energetic spectrum.** For women, this may manifest as disconnecting from assertiveness, sensuality, or agency. For men, it often means silencing vulnerability, surrender, and the need to be nurtured. For nonbinary and gender-expansive individuals, it may mean battling societal expectations that force binary alignment rather than allowing their full expression.

This internal conflict becomes an identity rupture. Clients often describe feeling like they are "performing" who they're expected to be while quietly yearning to express deeper truths. This incongruence leads to emotional exhaustion, poor boundaries, self-sabotage, and even somatic symptoms like fatigue, autoimmune flares, and hormonal instability.

> "Most of us are not broken—we are just stuck in a single polarity that no longer serves us." — Dr. Deilen Michelle Villegas

When we restore balance within, we show up differently in every relationship—with lovers, with children, with our own reflection in the mirror.

Clinical Insight

As clinicians, we must look beyond the surface-level symptoms and invite clients to explore:

- Which polarity do they default to under stress?

- Which polarity was safest to express in childhood?

- Where do they feel most alive: in structure or flow, action or surrender?

Healing polarity within identity is not about becoming "balanced" at all times. It's about restoring **choice**—the freedom to access the right energy for the right moment without shame or self-abandonment.

Mental Health Implications of Polarity Imbalance

Clinical research and therapeutic practice consistently reveal that **long-term disconnection from one's innate polarity—**

whether due to trauma, cultural programming, or chronic stress—can have significant implications for mental and physical health. Human beings are designed to operate with dynamic fluidity between assertive and receptive energies, but when survival or conditioning forces someone to over-identify with one end of the spectrum, **psychological rigidity and somatic distress** often follow.

Over-identification with traditionally *masculine* traits—such as hyper-productivity, stoicism, hyper-independence, and suppression of emotional vulnerability—can result in burnout, chronic stress, irritability, emotional detachment, and isolation. From a nervous system perspective, this is often linked to **persistent sympathetic activation**—the body remains in a low-grade state of fight-or-flight, even during rest.

Clients in this category may present with:

- Generalized anxiety or panic attacks

- Sleep disturbances

- Irritable bowel or gut-brain axis dysregulation

- Difficulty forming emotionally secure relationships

- Chronic dissatisfaction or performance-based self-worth

On the other end of the spectrum, over-reliance on *feminine* traits—such as over-nurturing, people-pleasing, emotional overexertion, and lack of boundaries—can manifest as **codependency, exhaustion, emotional instability, and autoimmune issues.** These clients may find themselves consistently absorbing the emotions of others while neglecting their own needs, resulting in chronic fatigue, adrenal burnout, and a diminished sense of agency.

> "When we silence our authentic polarity to survive,
> we fracture our psyche."
> — Dr. Gabor Maté (2003)

From a psychoneuroimmunological lens, polarity imbalance triggers **neuroendocrine disruption**: elevated cortisol, diminished oxytocin, impaired vagal tone, and altered levels of testosterone and estrogen. This internal biochemical chaos affects not just mood, but immune function, sexual health, memory, and long-term disease risk.

Case Insight: Emotional Collapse from Chronic Overfunctioning

Maya, a 41-year-old Latina entrepreneur and mother of two, came to therapy with symptoms of exhaustion, depression, and brain fog. Despite her professional success, she felt numb in her relationships and disconnected from joy. Upon mapping her energetic patterns, we discovered a strong overidentification with masculine polarity: always "on," managing everyone's needs, avoiding vulnerability, and struggling to ask for help.

Through nervous system regulation, inner child exploration, and a structured rest protocol, Maya began releasing the internalized belief that softness equaled weakness. She started weekly movement therapy sessions (dance and slow yoga), created sacred space for alone time, and began expressing emotional needs in her marriage. Within three months, her energy increased, libido returned, and her depressive symptoms significantly improved.

> The mind heals when the body is allowed to express
> what it has been holding in silence.

Healing Is About Recalibration, Not Extremes

The therapeutic goal is not to swing from one extreme to the other—it is to **restore functional emotional agility.** Healing polarity does not require one to discard either energy, but to reclaim the ability to choose. We do this by helping clients identify their **adaptive strategies** and gently reconnect to the parts of themselves that were exiled for survival.

Examples of Clinical Interventions:

- Breathwork and somatic tracking to access suppressed emotion or stored rage

- Art therapy or sacred movement to reconnect with pleasure and intuition

- Cognitive reframing and assertiveness training to re-establish healthy boundaries

- Hormone-friendly lifestyle shifts to support emotional regulation (adaptogens, blood sugar stability, movement rhythms)

Reflection for Clients:

- Where have I learned that I must suppress softness to be safe?

- What does "doing too much" cost me emotionally or physically?

- Am I afraid to be seen as too much or not enough?

- When do I feel most connected to myself—and what polarity am I in during those moments?

Practitioner Note: Always assess for trauma history when polarity imbalance is present. Often, chronic overfunctioning or emotional suppression began as a protective mechanism in early life—especially in households where one polarity (e.g., sensitivity or assertiveness) was punished, shamed, or neglected.

Clinical Tools for Balancing Polarity

Balancing polarity is not simply a cognitive task—it requires somatic integration, emotional safety, and neurobiological recalibration. The therapeutic goal is not to enforce a rigid model of masculine and feminine energies, but to support clients in **reclaiming disowned parts**, releasing adaptive survival strategies, and embodying authentic expression.

Below are foundational approaches that have proven effective in helping clients explore, integrate, and balance their internal polarity:

1. Somatic Experiencing® (SE): Reclaiming Safety in the Body

Developed by Dr. Peter Levine, Somatic Experiencing helps clients renegotiate trauma held in the body through **bottom-up processing**. Many polarity imbalances stem from unresolved trauma that forces the client into chronic sympathetic activation (fight/flight) or dorsal vagal shutdown (freeze/fawn).

Application for Polarity Work:

- Clients stuck in hyper-masculine states (overdrive, dissociation, control) can be guided into safe surrender, grounding, and receptivity through SE touchpoints.

- Clients overly fused with feminine energy (people-pleasing, emotional flooding, collapse) can be supported in titrating activation and reclaiming empowered boundary setting.

Practitioner Tool: Use pendulation (moving between sensation and safety) to help clients access states they avoid (e.g., anger, grief, softness, voice). Notice where masculine/feminine energies live in the body.

2. Parts Work / Internal Family Systems (IFS): Meeting the Inner Archetypes

IFS offers a profound framework to explore the **subpersonalities or "parts"** that govern behavior. Clients may have a protector part who suppresses their sensuality, or an inner child exiled for being "too loud," "too soft," or "too needy." These often map onto gendered or polarized roles.

Application for Polarity Work:

- Help clients identify their *"inner masculine"* and *"inner feminine"* parts and develop relationships with each.

- Guide clients to explore the burdens each part carries (e.g., "I must protect at all costs," "It's not safe to need others," "My worth is in my usefulness").

- Use guided imagery and somatic anchoring to allow parts to express, release, and integrate.

Client Example: One client, who was hyper-independent and emotionally shut down, discovered a fierce "warrior protector" part who was suppressing a deeply tender, intuitive artist. Integration allowed her to lead her business from creativity rather than control.

3. Narrative Therapy: Rewriting the Gendered Story

Clients often carry inherited narratives about what it means to be "a good woman," "a strong man," or "a person who belongs." These scripts are shaped by culture, religion, family, and systemic oppression. Narrative Therapy invites clients to become the **authors of their own story**.

Application for Polarity Work:

- Invite clients to externalize internalized roles (e.g., "the provider," "the caretaker," "the stoic," "the silent one").

- Deconstruct social and familial expectations around gendered behavior.

- Re-author new identities that embrace complexity: "I can be soft and powerful," "I can be sensual and spiritual," "I can lead and still receive."

Prompt: "What did you learn about who you're allowed to be? And who decides?"

4. Couples Counseling with Polarity Mapping

In relationships, polarity imbalance often leads to disconnection, communication breakdowns, and intimacy loss. When one partner chronically over-functions in one energy, the other may feel resentful, passive, or invisible.

Polarity Mapping Technique:

- Use a visual polarity spectrum (assertive/receptive, structured/flowing, direct/intuitive) to help partners see where each of them operates in different situations.

- Identify where roles have become rigid and where role reversal or flexibility is needed.

- Encourage conscious polarity play in intimacy (e.g., who initiates, who leads, who holds space, who receives).

Clinical Note: Healthy polarity creates *dynamic tension*, not power imbalance. The goal is energetic complementarity, not dominance.

Additional Tools & Practices:

- **Breathwork:** Use specific techniques to activate sympathetic (masculine) or parasympathetic (feminine) branches of the nervous system.

- **Embodiment Coaching:** Encourage movement practices that cultivate polarity—e.g., martial arts for masculine grounding, sensual dance for feminine flow.

- **Hormonal & Cycle Awareness:** Teach clients how hormonal shifts (e.g., luteal phase, testosterone peaks, adrenal fatigue) impact their energetic expression.

"When clients meet their inner masculine and feminine with compassion, they begin to embody wholeness."
— Dr. Deilen Michelle Villegas

Balancing polarity is a journey of **coming home to the body**, releasing performance-based identity, and learning to live from a place of wholeness rather than adaptation. When we offer clients tools for this reclamation, we do more than address symptoms—we awaken their truth.

Visual Aid: Polarity Spectrum Chart

Trait Spectrum	Masculine Polarity	Feminine Polarity
Decision-Making	Logical, Directive	Intuitive, Receptive
Communication	Succinct, Task-Oriented	Expressive, Emotion-Centered
Energy Focus	Goal-Driven, Structured	Flow-Oriented, Spontaneous
Emotional Response	Contained, Rationalized	Empathic, Relational
Sexual Expression	Penetrative, Assertive	Magnetic, Inviting

Embodying Integration

True healing unfolds not in the absence of polarity, but in the dance between its energies—when the masculine and feminine within are no longer at war, but in rhythm. Integration is the conscious embodiment of both structure and flow, logic and emotion, presence and passion. It is not a rigid balance, but a fluid state of wholeness that adapts moment to moment, experience to experience.

In clinical work, we often see clients struggle with internal fragmentation: the executive who cannot cry, the nurturer who cannot say no, the creative who cannot organize. These struggles are rarely about capacity; they are about permission. Integration offers that permission—to feel the full range of who we are without shame or suppression.

Embodying integration means:

- A woman can lead with assertiveness and still rest in softness.

- A man can protect and provide while also nurturing and receiving.

- A nonbinary individual can express dynamic shifts in energy without needing to conform to binaries society insists on.

- A clinician can bring structure into sessions while remaining deeply attuned and intuitive.

Integration is a **somatic experience**, not just a psychological insight. It's felt in the body—through breath, tone, posture, and presence. It is when your voice resonates from your gut *and* your heart. It is when decisions are both well-reasoned and soul-aligned. It's when touch, words, and boundaries all reflect a harmony within.

This chapter invites you, the reader, whether clinician or client, to begin noticing your inner polarities as gifts rather than contradictions. You are allowed to be both driven and delicate, focused and feeling, fierce and forgiving.

As practitioners, we must model this wholeness. Our presence teaches more than our interventions. When we show up integrated—comfortable with our power and our tenderness— we create safety for clients to do the same.

We are not here to enforce outdated gender scripts or diminish the sacred individuality of identity expression. We are here to **guide reconnection**: to body, to soul, and to the full spectrum of human expression that lives beyond binaries.

> "Healing is not about choosing one side of yourself over the other. It's about remembering you were never meant to live split."
> — Dr. Deilen Michelle Villegas

In the next chapter, we'll explore how these internal polarities shape and are shaped by **intimate relationships**, how **hormonal fluctuations** influence attraction and emotional regulation, and how the sacred tension of polarity can either enliven or erode connection over time.

References

Bangasser, D. A., & Cuarenta, A. (2021). Sex differences in anxiety and depression: Circuits and mechanisms. *Nature Reviews Neuroscience, 22*(7), 471–484. https://doi.org/10.1038/s41583-021-00461-0

Ingalhalikar, M., Smith, A., Parker, D., Satterthwaite, T. D., Elliott, M. A., Ruparel, K., ... & Verma, R. (2014). Sex differences in the structural connectome of the human brain. *Proceedings of the National Academy of Sciences, 111*(2), 823-828. https:// doi.org/10.1073/pnas.1316909110

Maté, G. (2003). *When the body says no: Exploring the stress-disease connection.* Wiley.

Porges, S. W. (2011). *The polyvagal theory: Neurophysiological foundations of emotions, attachment, communication, and self-regulation.* W. W. Norton & Company.

CHAPTER 2

Relationships & Hormonal Interplay

Love as a Biochemical Symphony

Love, intimacy, and connection are not just emotional experiences—they are *physiological events*. Our nervous systems, endocrine responses, and limbic circuitry co-create the experience of closeness, safety, and desire. The flutter in the chest, the feeling of "butterflies," the longing for connection, the comfort of touch—all of these are orchestrated by a powerful hormonal symphony that governs our human need for bonding and belonging.

In clinical settings, it becomes clear: unresolved trauma, hormonal imbalances, and nervous system dysregulation can profoundly interfere with one's ability to give or receive love. Couples often find themselves caught in patterns of misunderstanding, withdrawal, or hyper-reactivity—not due to lack of love, but due to dysregulated biology.

The Chemistry of Love

Love activates a precise sequence of hormonal and neurochemical activity:

- **Dopamine**, the neurotransmitter of reward, spikes during the early stages of attraction. It gives us that euphoric feeling of being "high" on love. It increases energy, motivation, and novelty-seeking behavior. But it can also create addiction to the highs of infatuation—often mistaken for genuine connection.

- **Oxytocin**, known as the "bonding hormone," is released through touch, eye contact, orgasm, and emotional intimacy. It cultivates trust, deepens attachment, and reduces stress. In relationships, oxytocin is a foundational element of long-term bonding and co-regulation.

- **Testosterone** and **estrogen** modulate sexual desire, drive, and energy. Testosterone fuels libido and assertive expression, while estrogen enhances emotional attunement and sensual pleasure. Both are essential in creating polarity and attraction within partnerships—regardless of gender.

- **Vasopressin**, another bonding hormone, supports monogamous pair bonding, protective behaviors, and long-term commitment. It also contributes to feelings of territoriality, which can manifest as possessiveness or jealousy when dysregulated.

- **Cortisol**, the stress hormone, can override all of the above. When the body is in chronic stress, love becomes less about bonding and more about survival. This is why trauma, unresolved emotional wounding, or constant overwhelm can sabotage even the most loving intentions.

"We fall in love through the heart, but we bond through the brain." – Dr. Deilen Michelle Villegas

Attachment Styles and Hormonal Roots

Attachment isn't just a psychological framework—it is a *neurobiological imprint* forged through early life experiences and biochemical patterns. People with anxious attachment often have heightened oxytocin sensitivity but lower baseline dopamine, driving them to seek validation and reassurance. Those with avoidant attachment may have lower oxytocin production and higher stress hormones, making intimacy feel unsafe.

Understanding these patterns allows clinicians and clients to reframe dysfunction in relationships not as character flaws, but as hormonal conditioning. This reframing reduces shame and opens the door to healing with compassion.

Sex, Safety, and the Nervous System

In trauma-informed somatic work, we emphasize that *safety is the precursor to pleasure*. For many clients, especially survivors of relational trauma, sexual touch can trigger a fight, flight, or freeze response. This occurs when oxytocin pathways are compromised or when the nervous system perceives closeness as a threat.

Sexual arousal requires a shift into parasympathetic dominance—a relaxed, open, receptive state. If someone is operating from sympathetic overdrive (chronic stress, anxiety, hypervigilance), they may struggle to feel desire or reach orgasm. Hormonal imbalances in estrogen, progesterone, or testosterone only compound this issue.

Case Study: Talia

Talia, a 36-year-old Latina client, reported a sharp decline in sexual desire after having her second child. Though she loved her husband deeply, every attempt at intimacy left her feeling "touched out" and emotionally distant. Lab tests revealed a drop in estrogen and oxytocin, coupled with elevated cortisol. Through integrative therapy—including pelvic breathwork, herbal adaptogens, nervous system tracking, and couples intimacy sessions—Talia began to restore her hormonal equilibrium. With time, her libido returned, not as a duty, but as a joyful, embodied desire.

Communication and Chemistry

Hormones influence not only our feelings of desire but our ability to communicate them. Estrogen enhances verbal fluency and empathy, while testosterone supports directness and boundary-setting. Couples often misinterpret these tendencies: a partner might perceive assertiveness as coldness, or emotional expressiveness as "too much." In truth, they're navigating biochemical differences that require *translation*, not judgment.

Hormonal literacy empowers couples to stop blaming and start *understanding*—creating the conditions for emotionally safe, sexually vibrant, and spiritually aligned partnerships.

Hormones and Attachment Styles

Attachment theory posits that our early childhood experiences form internal working models—mental blueprints of safety, love, and connection—that guide how we relate to others in adulthood. These attachment patterns are not purely psychological; they are deeply *biochemical*, rooted in the regulation and interplay of hormones that govern our sense of trust, safety, and belonging.

At the heart of secure attachment is **oxytocin**, the "bonding hormone." Oxytocin is released during breastfeeding, hugging, eye contact, orgasm, and moments of emotional vulnerability. It promotes feelings of closeness, empathy, and stress reduction. In secure attachment, individuals regulate oxytocin and **cortisol** more effectively, maintaining a nervous system that can recover from emotional stress and remain open to intimacy.

However, those with **anxious attachment** often have irregular oxytocin and dopamine patterns. They may experience overwhelming craving for connection, intense fear of abandonment, and difficulty soothing themselves when separated from a partner. Biochemically, this reflects a nervous system that is primed for hyperarousal—marked by elevated cortisol and impaired oxytocin response. Their bodies remain in a heightened state of alert, seeking safety through proximity and reassurance.

Conversely, individuals with **avoidant attachment** often have suppressed oxytocin and heightened vasopressin or cortisol activity. These individuals may feel emotionally overwhelmed by intimacy, preferring distance and independence. Their bodies have learned to regulate through withdrawal, not connection. In these cases, love and closeness may unconsciously signal threat, triggering a protective shutdown of bonding chemistry.

> "Attachment is not just about what happened in our past—it's about what our bodies learned to feel safe with." — Dr. Deilen Michelle Villegas

Vasopressin and Male Attachment

Another key player in adult attachment, especially in men, is **vasopressin**—a neuropeptide that contributes to pair bonding, protective instincts, and territorial behavior. Animal studies on prairie voles, one of the few monogamous species, revealed that differences in vasopressin receptor distribution correlate with whether males form lifelong pair bonds or remain solitary (Lim & Young, 2006). In humans, variations in vasopressin receptor genes have been linked to relationship satisfaction, fidelity, and emotional availability.

When vasopressin is in balance, it fosters loyalty, long-term bonding, and an invested interest in a partner's wellbeing. When dysregulated, it may contribute to emotional detachment, jealousy, or relational apathy. In men who experienced early attachment trauma or were raised in emotionally neglectful environments, vasopressin signaling may be altered—making commitment or sustained emotional presence more difficult.

Importantly, this insight shifts the narrative: *intimacy issues are not always rooted in character flaws*. Many clients internalize guilt or shame for struggling to bond, commit, or remain emotionally available. But what appears as relational dysfunction may, in fact, be a neurochemical response shaped by trauma, neglect, or survival adaptation.

Clinical Implications

Understanding the hormonal underpinnings of attachment allows clinicians to tailor interventions that go beyond talk therapy and directly support the client's physiological capacity for connection:

- **For anxious attachment**: Practices that stabilize the nervous system (e.g., vagal toning, breathwork, co-regulation exercises) can support oxytocin and lower cortisol.

- **For avoidant attachment**: Gentle somatic work and safe emotional exposure may increase oxytocin tolerance and reduce the threat response to intimacy.

- **For disorganized attachment**: Trauma-informed interventions that focus on establishing safety, consistent attunement, and rebuilding trust in bodily cues are essential.

Hormonal literacy also allows couples to reframe their struggles with compassion. A partner who withdraws during conflict may not be cold—they may be flooded. A partner who clings tightly may not be needy—they may be afraid of abandonment wired into their very biology.

Practical Tools: Harmonizing the Hormonal Symphony

- **Couples Polarity Mapping**: Identify dominant energetic/hormonal tendencies and how they interact under stress and intimacy.

- **Pre-Intimacy Rituals**: Breathwork, eye-gazing, or shared meditation to regulate oxytocin and reduce cortisol.

- **Cycle Awareness**: Teach partners how menstrual, hormonal, or adrenal cycles influence libido, emotion, and energy.

- **Adaptogenic Support**: Herbs like maca, ashwagandha, and rhodiola to balance cortisol and support reproductive hormones.

- **Sleep, Touch, and Trust**: Encourage physical affection outside of sex, prioritizing co-regulation and comfort.

The Dopamine Cycle of Desire

Desire is not just an emotion—it's a biochemical symphony, orchestrated by the ebb and flow of neurotransmitters and hormones. At the center of this cycle is **dopamine**, the neurotransmitter of anticipation, novelty, and reward.

In the initial stages of attraction—what many call the "honeymoon phase"—dopamine floods the brain, particularly in the **mesolimbic reward pathway**. This neurochemical high mirrors the brain's response to stimulants like cocaine, producing feelings of euphoria, infatuation, and tunnel-visioned focus on the object of desire (Fisher, 2004). It explains why new lovers lose track of time, feel more alive, and become temporarily obsessed with each other.

However, **this phase is neurochemically unsustainable**. Over time, the brain downregulates dopamine sensitivity to return to baseline. When this happens, partners may mistake the natural decline in intensity as boredom, incompatibility, or even "falling out of love." In reality, the body is simply asking for a shift—from dopamine-driven infatuation to **oxytocin-**

based bonding and **vasopressin-rooted loyalty**.

This transition can create friction in relationships—especially when one partner is addicted to novelty and the other craves predictability. If unaddressed, this mismatch can lead to withdrawal, affairs, or chronic dissatisfaction.

> "Love begins with dopamine, but it deepens with oxytocin. Desire is a flame—connection is the hearth." — Dr. Deilen Michelle Villegas

Why Understanding the Cycle Matters

Couples often arrive in therapy believing the "spark is gone," when in truth, they've hit the **dopamine dip**—a natural lull that calls for reorientation, not resignation.

This dip doesn't mean desire is dead; it means desire must evolve.

Educating couples on this **neurochemical shift**:

- Reduces shame and blame

- Validates the reality of changing desire

- Empowers conscious partnership

- Opens the door to rekindling intimacy through presence, not pressure

Case Study: Alina and Marcus

Alina (33) and **Marcus (37)**, seven years into marriage, presented with what they called "a lost spark." Marcus expressed growing resentment that Alina no longer initiated physical intimacy. Alina, in contrast, reported feeling emotionally abandoned and physically overwhelmed by her roles as a mother, caretaker, and household manager.

Upon assessment:

- Alina showed signs of **adrenal dysregulation**: elevated cortisol, suppressed progesterone, irregular sleep, and low libido.

- Marcus, often traveling for work, showed subtle signs of **testosterone fluctuation** and reduced vasopressin engagement—likely due to stress and relational disconnection.

Despite still loving one another, their **dopamine cycle had stalled**. Their intimacy was not broken—it was **overstimulated, undernourished, and unregulated**.

Their therapeutic roadmap included:

- **Oxytocin rituals**: Daily non-sexual touch (shoulder rubs, hand-holding, eye contact), to rebuild safety and trust.

- **Adrenal and sleep support** for Alina: Magnesium, ashwagandha, progesterone-boosting foods, and a consistent wind-down ritual.

- **Scheduled intimacy**: Not performance-based, but rooted in presence, slow sensuality, and mutual care.

- **Emotional mapping sessions**: Each partner shared unmet emotional needs without judgment, fostering emotional vulnerability and co-regulation.

Over time, their intimacy didn't just "return"—it *transformed*. With their nervous systems no longer in survival mode, desire became a conscious practice rather than a fleeting feeling. The reestablishment of **neurochemical trust** restored both their physical and emotional closeness.

Therapeutic Takeaway

When couples understand that sexual desire fluctuates in cycles—not failures—they are less likely to pathologize their relationship. Instead, they learn to adapt, attune, and evolve their connection:

- **Desire is not always spontaneous—it is often cultivated.**

- **Intimacy is not a spark—it is a skill.**

- **Passion is not dead—it's dormant in nervous systems that no longer feel safe.**

Couples who make this transition move from hormone-driven highs to embodied, sustainable love.

Hormones and Communication Styles

Communication is not just a learned behavior—it is deeply influenced by the biochemical environment of the brain and body. The way we speak, listen, interpret tone, and engage in dialogue is shaped, in part, by our **hormonal landscape**, particularly levels of **testosterone** and **estrogen**.

Testosterone is associated with traits such as assertiveness, goal orientation, and solution-focused thinking. Individuals with higher testosterone—regardless of gender—may gravitate toward **direct, succinct, and action-driven** language. They tend to prioritize efficiency over emotional elaboration and may become frustrated by what they perceive as "circular" or emotionally layered conversations.

Estrogen, on the other hand, supports **verbal fluency, emotional expression, and empathic attunement** (Brizendine, 2006). Higher estrogen levels correlate with increased activity in brain regions associated with social bonding and language processing. This often results in a more **contextual, relational, and emotionally rich** communication style.

When these hormonal influences intersect in relationships —romantic, familial, or professional—they can either create **magnetic polarity** or lead to misunderstanding and misattunement. For example, one partner may interpret the other's problem-solving approach as dismissive, while the other sees emotional storytelling as unproductive. These are not character flaws—they are often **hormonal defaults**.

Hormonal Polarity in Dialogue

Rather than forcing individuals to conform to one "ideal" way of communicating, therapeutic work should explore and **honor their natural polarity** while supporting greater range and flexibility. This involves helping clients develop tools that balance their dominant communication tendencies:

For high-estrogen clients:

- Encourage **concise expression** when navigating conflict or boundary-setting.

- Practice **assertive communication frameworks** (e.g., "I feel... I need..." statements).

- Explore how emotional nuance can be a strength without becoming over-explaining or self-sacrificing.

For high-testosterone clients:

- Develop **emotional literacy** through feelings identification charts, body mapping, or journaling.

- Practice **active listening** skills—such as mirroring, summarizing, and asking clarifying questions.

- Encourage slowing down to allow **emotional data** to be processed, especially during relational tension.

Clinical Example: Gender Dynamics in Dialogue

In a couples session, **Jasmine (29)** expressed frustration that her partner, **Devin (31)**, "never really listens." Devin, in turn, felt overwhelmed by Jasmine's desire to "process every emotion."

A closer look at their hormonal and behavioral profiles revealed:

- Jasmine had **elevated estrogen and oxytocin sensitivity**, making her more attuned to tone, subtle cues, and emotional language.

- Devin, with **higher testosterone and cortisol**, favored quick resolutions and often shut down during emotionally charged conversations.

Their therapeutic intervention focused on:

- Jasmine learning to **ground her emotions before initiating dialogue**, using breathwork and journaling.

- Devin practicing **non-defensive listening**, repeating back what he heard, and checking in emotionally before offering solutions.

With practice, their once-oppositional styles became **complementary**. Jasmine appreciated Devin's steadiness, and Devin began to value the depth and insight Jasmine brought to their relationship.

Energetic Communication Patterns

Beyond hormones, communication styles also reflect **masculine and feminine energetic patterns**:

- **Masculine communication** seeks clarity, direction, and purpose.

- **Feminine communication** seeks connection, empathy, and emotional depth.

Both are valuable. Integration occurs when an individual can move fluidly between both—offering assertiveness with compassion, or empathy with clarity, depending on the moment.

Therapeutic Application

Use communication polarity mapping to help clients:

- Recognize their default patterns under stress

- Identify where communication breakdowns occur

- Explore new patterns that foster both expression and attunement

"Hormones influence our words, but healing transforms our conversations." — Dr. Villegas

Chart: Hormonal Influence on Relationship Behavior

Hormone	Influences	Imbalance Effects
Oxytocin	Bonding, trust, nurturing	Anxiety, detachment, fear of closeness
Dopamine	Desire, novelty, motivation	Addiction, dissatisfaction, boredom
Cortisol	Stress regulation	Burnout, irritability, conflict reactivity
Estrogen	Emotional fluency, connection	Oversensitivity, mood swings

Testosterone	Confidence, libido, focus	Aggression, withdrawal, low motivation

Clinical Integration

Hormonal harmony is not only a matter of internal balance —it is the unseen infrastructure of our relationships. When our hormones are dysregulated, our ability to connect, communicate, and remain emotionally present is compromised. Therefore, **therapeutic strategies that target both biochemical regulation and relational repair** are essential.

Below are key integrative approaches that practitioners can use to rebalance relationship hormones and create more connected, embodied partnerships:

1. Touch Therapy: Oxytocin Activation

Intentional, non-sexual touch—such as **hand-holding, skin-to-skin contact, or gentle massage**—stimulates the release of **oxytocin**, the hormone responsible for bonding, emotional trust, and feelings of safety.

Oxytocin counters cortisol, soothing the nervous system and reinforcing secure attachment. In couples therapy, guiding partners through structured touch exercises (e.g., "30-second hugs" or "mirror holding") can **rekindle connection without the pressure of performance.**

> **Clinical note**: This is especially powerful for partners with trauma histories who may fear intimacy but crave closeness.

2. Adaptogenic Herbs & Nutritional Support: Cortisol Modulation

Chronic stress and adrenal fatigue can suppress libido, empathy, and connection. Elevated **cortisol levels** blunt the release of oxytocin, disrupt progesterone production, and desensitize dopamine receptors—leaving clients feeling disconnected, irritable, or emotionally flat.

Therapeutic nutrition and **adaptogenic herbs** such as *ashwagandha*, *rhodiola*, *maca*, and *holy basil* can help restore adrenal balance. Coupled with sleep hygiene and blood sugar regulation, these interventions provide the **biological foundation for emotional intimacy to thrive**.

> **Pro tip**: Recommend clients track their energy and mood throughout the menstrual or hormonal cycle to tailor nutritional and herbal strategies accordingly.

3. Erotic Blueprint Exploration: Shame-Free Dopamine Engagement

Desire is not only emotional—it is **neurochemical**. Many clients operate from a place of **dopaminergic depletion**, meaning they lack novelty, pleasure, and reward in their intimate lives. This often leads to shame, avoidance, or infidelity.

Introducing the concept of **Erotic Blueprints** (sensual, energetic, kinky, sexual, and shapeshifter) allows clients to explore their unique erotic language without judgment. This taps into **dopamine and oxytocin** pathways, reinvigorating desire and pleasure without external pressure.

> "Understanding your Erotic Blueprint is like unlocking your nervous system's personal pleasure code."

4. Mindfulness-Based Intimacy: Enhancing Presence & Parasympathetic Tone

Mindful presence is one of the most powerful tools for relational healing. Practices such as **eye gazing, synchronized breathing, and tantric touch** bring partners into **co-regulation**, where heart rate, breath, and brainwaves synchronize.

This activates the **parasympathetic nervous system**, downregulates cortisol, and opens the doorway to **safe vulnerability**. Clients learn to communicate not just with words, but with presence.

> Use **body scans, somatic tracking, or guided visualization** to help clients drop into their body and out of reactive states.

Integrated Case Application:

A couple presents in therapy reporting "low libido" and "communication breakdown." Rather than labeling this as a relationship issue alone, you assess the **hormonal and nervous system context**:

- One partner is experiencing adrenal burnout, high cortisol, and estrogen dominance.

- The other has low dopamine engagement and avoidant intimacy patterns.

Your therapeutic plan includes:

- Touch-based oxytocin exercises

- Adaptogenic and nutrition support

- Erotic blueprint exploration to reintroduce play and novelty

- Breathwork and body-based communication to restore presence

Within weeks, they begin to **feel seen, safe, and sexually alive** again—not because of talk therapy alone, but because their

biology was brought into the conversation.

"Hormones don't make relationships work—but they do shape the landscape we try to navigate them on." — Dr. Deilen Michelle Villegas

Conscious Chemistry in Connection

Healthy relationships aren't sustained by emotion alone —they're upheld by **embodied awareness**, **biochemical attunement**, and a shared commitment to growth. While love, attraction, and compatibility may spark the flame, it is **conscious chemistry**—the interplay of regulated nervous systems, hormonal balance, and intentional communication —that keeps it burning.

At the heart of every thriving relationship is **nervous system co-regulation**. When both partners can stay present during stress, conflict, or intimacy, their physiological signals —heartbeat, breath, and tone—sync up to create safety. This biological safety net fosters **emotional vulnerability**, strengthens trust, and allows desire to be expressed without fear or performance.

But when one or both individuals are living in chronic dysregulation—high cortisol, low dopamine, unprocessed trauma—the relationship can feel like emotional whiplash. Arguments escalate, touch feels overwhelming or disconnected, and partners may confuse biological stress signals for incompatibility or emotional failure.

Understanding that **"it's not always personal—it's chemical"** is a revolutionary concept in therapy. When clients learn that:

- A dip in progesterone might be why they feel tearful or irritable

- A testosterone crash may be behind their partner's emotional distance

- Elevated cortisol from work stress can shut down sexual desire

They begin to shift from **blame to curiosity**, from reactivity to responsibility.

This awareness creates a **third space** in the relationship: one that honors both the emotional and biological truths. In this space, couples can learn:

- How to pause during conflict to regulate breath and nervous system before speaking

- How to touch in ways that release oxytocin and restore felt safety

- How to support each other nutritionally and hormonally through life's seasons and cycles

- How to cultivate erotic polarity even amidst daily stressors

Conscious chemistry also invites a deeper spiritual and energetic alignment—where intimacy becomes **a mirror**, revealing where love lives freely and where wounds still ask for healing.

> "Love is not just what we feel. It's how we choose to regulate, repair, and rise together."

In therapy, this shifts the paradigm from **pathology to partnership**. Instead of seeing emotional distance, low libido, or tension as signs of failure, couples begin to see them as invitations to deepen, heal, and rebalance.

In the next chapter, we'll dive into the **individual hormonal blueprints** that shape these patterns—beginning with **estrogen, progesterone, and testosterone**—their physiological roles, behavioral influences, and the ripple effects of imbalance on mood, intimacy, and identity.

References

Brizendine, L. (2006). *The female brain.* Morgan Road Books.

Fisher, H. E. (2004). *Why we love: The nature and chemistry of romantic love.* Henry Holt and Company.

Lim, M. M., & Young, L. J. (2006). Neuropeptidergic regulation of affiliative behavior and social bonding in animals. *Hormones and Behavior, 50*(4), 506–517. https://doi.org/10.1016/j.yhbeh.2006.06.028

Ziegler, T. E. (2021). Hormones and human social behavior. *Current Opinion in Psychology, 43*, 121–127. https://doi.org/10.1016/j.copsyc.2021.07.004

CHAPTER 3

Estrogen, Progesterone & Testosterone – Foundations & Imbalances

The Hormonal Triad of Life

Hormones are not just background players in the human body—they are the **conductors of our internal orchestra**, influencing everything from our metabolism and mood to libido, brain function, emotional resilience, and relational harmony. Of the many hormones circulating through our system, **estrogen, progesterone, and testosterone** form the foundational triad. These three act not only as chemical messengers, but as **energetic translators**—turning our thoughts, stress, desires, and nourishment into physiological action.

Though traditionally classified as "female" or "male" hormones, this triad exists in all people, regardless of sex or gender identity. Their **relative ratios, sensitivity of receptor sites**, and **timing of release** are what create differences in expression. The goal of hormonal healing is not to eliminate these differences, but to **understand them**—and to support optimal harmony, especially during periods of natural transition (puberty, postpartum, perimenopause, and andropause).

> "Hormonal balance is less about having more or less —and more about having the right rhythm for your body's unique needs." — Dr. Villegas

Estrogen: The Architect of Growth and Sensitivity

Estrogen is not simply a "female hormone"—it is a master communicator that orchestrates growth, reproduction, vascular health, bone density, mood regulation, and neuroplasticity. It plays a central role in how individuals relate, feel, and adapt to their environment, making it both a biological and emotional architect. Produced primarily in the ovaries for women, and in smaller amounts by the testes and adrenal glands in men, estrogen exists in several forms —**estradiol (E2), estrone (E1), and estriol (E3)**—each with distinct functions and potencies.

Estrogen receptors are widespread throughout the body: in the brain, bones, breasts, uterus, blood vessels, and even the skin. This wide reach explains why estrogen imbalances can affect such a vast array of systems—manifesting not just as menstrual irregularities, but as cognitive fog, emotional dysregulation, or cardiovascular concerns.

The Power and Sensitivity of Estrogen

Estrogen enhances:

- **Synaptic communication in the brain**, boosting memory and learning capacity

- **Serotonin production and receptor sensitivity**, supporting mood regulation and resilience to stress

- **Vaginal tissue integrity and lubrication**, contributing to comfort during intimacy

- **Skin elasticity and collagen production**, preserving youthful appearance

- **Vascular flexibility**, offering cardioprotective effects before menopause

- **Bone remodeling**, reducing the risk of osteoporosis

Because of its broad influence, fluctuations in estrogen

—especially during perimenopause, postpartum, or due to chronic stress—can lead to symptoms that mimic mental health conditions such as anxiety, depression, and even panic disorders.

Signs of High Estrogen (Often Paired with Low Progesterone)

- **Mood swings**, especially premenstrually

- **Breast tenderness** or swelling

- **Water retention and bloating**

- **Weight gain**, particularly in the hips and thighs

- **Heavy or painful periods**

- **Fibroids, endometriosis, or endometrial thickening**

- **Headaches or migraines**

- **Irritability or heightened emotional sensitivity**

This state, often called **estrogen dominance**, does not always mean estrogen is objectively high—it may simply be out of balance with low progesterone. Chronic exposure to **xenoestrogens** (synthetic compounds that mimic estrogen in the body) contributes significantly to this imbalance. These are found in:

- Plastic containers (especially when heated)

- Non-organic meat and dairy (due to hormone residues)

- Pesticide-laden produce

- Personal care products with parabens and phthalates

Signs of Low Estrogen

- **Vaginal dryness** and painful intercourse

- **Low libido**

- **Hot flashes and night sweats**

- **Insomnia or disrupted sleep cycles**

- **Depressed mood or emotional flatness**

- **Decreased concentration or memory fog**

- **Loss of skin elasticity and hair thinning**

- **Increased risk for bone fractures**

Estrogen levels often drop dramatically during **perimenopause and menopause**, but they can also dip due to extreme stress, disordered eating, excessive exercise, or after hysterectomy or chemotherapy. Men may also experience a relative estrogen deficiency with aging or low testosterone, affecting mood, bone health, and libido.

Clinical Insight: Detoxification and Rebalancing

The **liver** is responsible for metabolizing and excreting excess estrogen through specific pathways (Phase I and Phase II detox). When the liver is overburdened by alcohol, processed food, environmental toxins, or chronic stress, estrogen clearance is impaired—leading to **recirculation** of unprocessed estrogen in the body.

Key support strategies include:

- **Cruciferous vegetables** (broccoli, cauliflower, Brussels sprouts) for DIM (diindolylmethane)

- **Calcium-D-glucarate** to support glucuronidation (liver detox pathway)

- **Adequate fiber** to bind estrogen and facilitate excretion through stool

- **Sweating and hydration** to enhance elimination

- **Reducing xenoestrogen exposure** (glass containers, clean skincare, filtered water)

Integrative Approaches to Estrogen Balance

- **Herbal Support:** Chasteberry (Vitex), black cohosh, red clover, and rhodiola may help regulate estrogen cycles and alleviate symptoms.

- **Stress Regulation:** Chronic cortisol elevation suppresses ovarian function and can disrupt estrogen production. Nervous system regulation practices (e.g., vagal toning, breathwork) support overall endocrine health.

- **Functional Labs:** Salivary or Dutch hormone testing can help clinicians evaluate estrogen levels across the day and assess estrogen metabolism patterns.

"Estrogen teaches us that power and sensitivity are not opposites—they are partners in a delicate dance of balance."

— Dr. Deilen Michelle Villegas, Ph.D.

Progesterone: The Calming Counterbalance

Progesterone is the unsung hero of hormonal harmony—a natural mood stabilizer and physiological buffer that softens the sharp edges of life's daily stressors. Produced primarily in the ovaries after ovulation (during the luteal phase of the menstrual cycle) and in smaller amounts by the adrenal glands, progesterone plays a vital role in everything from fertility to neuroregulation.

Known as the "peacekeeper hormone," progesterone counterbalances estrogen's stimulating effects by activating calming neurotransmitter systems, reducing inflammation, supporting uterine lining health, and preparing the body for pregnancy. Its presence is crucial not only for conception and gestation but for mental and emotional equilibrium in menstruating and non-menstruating individuals alike.

Key Functions of Progesterone:

- **Supports implantation and pregnancy** by stabilizing the endometrium and preventing uterine contractions

- **Regulates GABA (gamma-aminobutyric acid)** receptors in the brain, which promote a sense of calm, reduce anxiety, and improve sleep quality

- **Reduces systemic inflammation**, aiding in immune modulation and reducing autoimmune flare-ups

- **Counters estrogen dominance**, preventing excessive tissue proliferation and emotional volatility

- **Protects brain function** by acting as a neurosteroid—especially important in perimenopausal and menopausal women

Because progesterone levels rise only after ovulation, any disruption in ovulation—whether from stress, aging, or metabolic imbalance—can lead to suboptimal levels. In this sense, **progesterone is not just a hormone—it's a barometer of how well a body is managing safety, stress, and balance.**

Signs of Low Progesterone:

- **Premenstrual anxiety or insomnia**

- **Irritability or mood swings**, particularly in the days leading up to menstruation

- **Spotting between periods** or short luteal phases (<10 days)

- **Difficulty conceiving**, especially from poor implantation

- **Recurrent miscarriages**

- **Headaches, especially hormonal migraines**

- **Breast tenderness or cysts**

- **Symptoms of estrogen dominance** (heavy periods, bloating, weight gain in hips/thighs)

Women in their mid-30s may begin to experience **a gradual decline in progesterone production**, even when estrogen remains relatively stable. This creates a **relative estrogen dominance**, where the calming influence of progesterone is no longer enough to buffer estrogen's stimulating effects—leading to irritability, sleeplessness, and heightened emotional reactivity.

Stress and the Progesterone-Cortisol Trade-Off

One of the most common causes of low progesterone in modern women is **chronic stress**. The body converts **pregnenolone**, the precursor hormone needed for progesterone, into **cortisol** during periods of prolonged stress—creating a biochemical tug-of-war known as the

"pregnenolone steal." When cortisol production takes priority, progesterone suffers, and the nervous system becomes increasingly dysregulated.

> *"You can't be calm and in crisis at the same time. The body will always prioritize survival over serenity."* — Dr. Deilen Michelle Villegas

This means even if a woman's ovulation is technically occurring, her **luteal phase** may be compromised, resulting in insufficient progesterone and subclinical symptoms that affect sleep, anxiety levels, or fertility.

Clinical Strategies for Rebalancing Progesterone:

1. Stress Regulation and Nervous System Support

- **Somatic tools**, breathwork, and vagal toning practices help reduce cortisol levels, freeing up resources for progesterone production.

- **Mindfulness and restorative sleep** are non-negotiable when it comes to progesterone recovery.

2. Targeted Nutritional Support

- **Magnesium**: Helps regulate cortisol and supports GABA production.

- **Vitamin B6**: Cofactor in progesterone synthesis.

- **Zinc**: Supports luteal phase function and balances estrogen.

- **Healthy fats (omega-3s, avocados, olive oil)**: Crucial for steroid hormone production.

3. Herbal and Functional Medicine Approaches

- **Chasteberry (Vitex agnus-castus)**: Supports luteinizing hormone (LH) production, which enhances ovulation and progesterone output.

- **Ashwagandha, Rhodiola, and Holy Basil**: Adaptogens that lower cortisol and restore hormonal resilience.

- **Evening Primrose Oil**: Can support luteal phase balance, especially in cases of premenstrual tension or irregular cycles.

4. Lifestyle Adjustments

- Reduce caffeine and alcohol, both of which can impair hormonal balance.

- Prioritize blood sugar stability (low progesterone is worsened by insulin spikes).

- Avoid overtraining and chronic cardio, which disrupt ovulation and increase cortisol.

Case Study: "Sofia"

Sofia, a 36-year-old Afro-Latina entrepreneur, presented with severe PMS, anxiety, and insomnia that worsened during the second half of her cycle. Labs revealed low luteal progesterone and elevated evening cortisol. She reported high work stress, skipped meals, and nighttime phone use.

Her holistic plan included:

- Daily magnesium glycinate and B6 supplementation

- Transitioning her evening routine to include blue light reduction and nervous system downregulation (yoga nidra and lavender oil)

- Introducing Vitex tincture during days 14–28 of her

cycle

- Adding nutrient-dense whole foods and blood sugar balancing snacks

After three months, Sofia reported improved sleep, shorter PMS duration, and decreased emotional reactivity. Her follow-up labs confirmed improved progesterone levels.

"Progesterone is your body's built-in exhale. When it's present, you feel safe enough to soften, rest, and receive."

— Dr. Deilen Michelle Villegas, Ph.D.

Testosterone: Power, Drive, and Direction

Often misunderstood and unfairly reduced to stereotypes of aggression or dominance, **testosterone** is far more than a "male hormone." It is a life force hormone—deeply connected to vitality, motivation, sexual drive, and executive function in **all bodies**, regardless of gender.

Produced primarily in the testes for men and in the ovaries and adrenal glands for women, testosterone plays a central role in:

- **Energy metabolism**

- **Cognitive clarity**

- **Mood regulation**

- **Libido**

- **Muscle development**

- **Confidence and assertiveness**

- **Bone strength and regeneration**

When in balance, testosterone fosters a grounded sense of presence, direction, and inner authority. When out of balance, it can contribute to mood dysregulation, fatigue, and identity disruption.

Signs of Low Testosterone (Across Genders):

- Persistent **fatigue or apathy**

- **Low libido** or difficulty reaching orgasm

- **Loss of strength** or difficulty building muscle

- **Increased body fat**, particularly around the midsection

- **Mood changes**, including depression, irritability, or low self-confidence

- **Erectile dysfunction** or decreased spontaneous erections in men

- **Brain fog**, decreased concentration, or forgetfulness

Signs of High Testosterone:

- **Acne or oily skin**, especially in the jawline or back

- **Excess facial or body hair** in women (hirsutism)

- **Scalp hair thinning** or male-pattern baldness

- **Irregular menstrual cycles**

- **Polycystic ovarian syndrome (PCOS)**—characterized by anovulation, cysts, insulin resistance, and elevated androgens

- **Increased aggression, impulsivity**, or mood swings

Modern Triggers of Testosterone Dysregulation

Testosterone levels are declining globally at an alarming rate, particularly among men under 40. This phenomenon —sometimes referred to as the **"Testosterone Recession"**— is fueled by a mix of environmental, nutritional, and psychosocial stressors:

- **Endocrine-disrupting chemicals (EDCs)** such as BPA, phthalates, and parabens found in plastics, canned food linings, personal care products, and pesticides

- **Chronic stress**, which elevates cortisol and suppresses testosterone synthesis

- **Sleep deprivation**, especially reduction in REM and deep sleep cycles

- **Sedentary lifestyle** and low muscle engagement

- **Poor nutrition**, especially diets high in processed foods and low in zinc, magnesium, and healthy fats

- **Metabolic syndrome and insulin resistance**, both of which lower testosterone production

- **Overtraining or excessive endurance exercise**, which leads to hormonal burnout and adrenal dysregulation

Women and Testosterone: The Missing Link in Energy & Desire

Testosterone plays a vital, yet often overlooked, role in female vitality. Low levels can result in:

- **Diminished sexual desire**

- **Poor orgasmic response**

- **Decreased competitive drive or ambition**

- **Emotional flatness**

- **Perimenopausal fatigue and bone loss**

Women naturally have lower levels of testosterone than men, but even small shifts in this hormone can profoundly affect **mood, libido, and energy**.

> "Testosterone is the spark that ignites motivation—
> not just for sex, but for life."
> — Dr. Deilen Michelle Villegas, Ph.D.

In conditions like PCOS, elevated testosterone contributes to physical and emotional challenges—but these increases are often rooted in insulin resistance and inflammation, not true androgen dominance. Understanding the **root cause** is essential for proper treatment.

Clinical Diagnostics and Testing

Functional medicine practitioners often assess testosterone using:

- **DUTCH Testing**: Tracks daily hormone patterns and metabolite conversion rates (including testosterone → DHT)

- **Salivary hormone panels**: Offer insight into bioavailable testosterone and its circadian rhythm

- **Serum labs**: Total and free testosterone levels, SHBG (sex hormone-binding globulin), and DHEA

Evaluating **testosterone in context**—alongside estrogen, progesterone, cortisol, and DHEA—gives a more accurate picture of what's really driving imbalance.

Rebalancing Testosterone Naturally

Lifestyle and Nutritional Interventions:

- **Strength training & resistance exercise**: Boosts natural testosterone production and improves receptor sensitivity

- **Quality sleep**: 7–9 hours of uninterrupted sleep is essential for testosterone synthesis

- **Healthy fats**: Avocados, grass-fed meats, olive oil, and nuts support hormone creation

- **Key nutrients**: Zinc, magnesium, vitamin D3, omega-3s, and boron

- **Blood sugar balance**: Reduces insulin resistance and improves testosterone stability

Botanical Support:

- **Ashwagandha**: Adaptogen that reduces cortisol and supports testosterone

- **Tongkat Ali (Longjack)**: Increases free testosterone and reduces stress-related suppression

- **Maca root**: Enhances libido and mood, particularly in women

- **Nettle root**: Supports free testosterone by inhibiting SHBG binding

Case Study: Jalen

Jalen, a 29-year-old Black man, came to counseling with symptoms of low motivation, mild depression, and decreased libido. Though physically active, he had recently gained abdominal weight and reported poor sleep due to late-night screen use and work stress. Labs showed **low free testosterone** and elevated **evening cortisol**.

His holistic treatment plan included:

- Replacing evening screens with wind-down breathwork and blue light blocking

- Strength-based workouts 4x/week and nature walks

- Nutritional support with zinc, magnesium, and adaptogens

- Mind-body coaching to address internalized pressure around masculinity and performance

After eight weeks, Jalen reported improved focus, increased morning erections, reduced anxiety, and a greater sense of personal confidence—evidence of hormonal and nervous system synergy.

Case Study: Layla and the Puzzle of Fatigue

Layla, a 29-year-old Latina client, presented with chronic fatigue, anxiety, low libido, and heavy periods. She had been prescribed SSRIs but reported emotional numbing without relief. Lab results showed low progesterone and high estrogen. A protocol was initiated that included nervous system support, targeted supplementation, liver detoxification, and cycle syncing practices.

Within three months, Layla experienced improved energy,

emotional resilience, and regular cycles. Understanding her hormonal landscape allowed her to reclaim agency and build a rhythm that supported—not silenced—her body.

"Masculinity is not measured in volume of testosterone, but in the harmony of energy, direction, and self-knowing. Balanced testosterone gives men and women the fire to create, protect, and lead—from a place of clarity, not chaos."

— Dr. Deilen Michelle Villegas

Visual: Hormonal Functions & Imbalance Matrix

Hormone	Primary Roles	High Levels May Cause	Low Levels May Cause
Estrogen	Reproduction, bone health, mood	PMS, fibroids, weight gain	Dryness, depression, bone loss
Progesterone	Calming, implantation, sleep regulation	Rare (sedation, bloating)	Anxiety, sleep issues, fertility problems
Testosterone	Libido, motivation, muscle building	Acne, aggression, PCOS	Fatigue, depression, low libido

Clinical Applications

Hormonal healing requires a multifaceted and individualized approach. Because hormones are sensitive to every input—from food and thoughts to trauma and relationships—effective treatment plans must address the full landscape of a client's internal and external environment. It is not enough to supplement deficiencies or suppress symptoms; true healing means **rebalancing the entire ecosystem of the body, mind, and nervous system.**

1. Functional Lab Testing: Precision Diagnostics for Personalized Care

Understanding a client's hormonal state begins with accurate data. Functional lab testing provides a deeper, more nuanced view than conventional bloodwork alone.

- **DUTCH Test (Dried Urine Test for Comprehensive Hormones):**
  Offers insights into sex hormone metabolites, cortisol rhythms, DHEA levels, and pathways of hormone detoxification. It also reveals how the body is metabolizing estrogen and whether it's shunting testosterone into DHT (a more potent androgen).

- **Saliva Testing:**
  Useful for assessing diurnal cortisol patterns, free (bioavailable) hormone levels, and circadian dysregulation.

- **Serum Blood Testing:**
  Ideal for tracking total hormone levels, thyroid panels, and nutrient deficiencies that affect hormone production (e.g., vitamin D, B12, magnesium, zinc, and iron).

Lab interpretation should go beyond "normal ranges" and focus on **optimal ranges** tailored to the client's sex, age, stage of life, and presenting symptoms.

2. Herbal and Nutritional Support: Rooted in Nature, Backed by Science

Once hormone imbalances are identified, **targeted herbal and nutritional interventions** can provide powerful support without harsh pharmaceuticals.

- **Adaptogens** (Ashwagandha, Rhodiola, Maca): Regulate cortisol, boost resilience to stress, and support hormonal harmony.

- **Liver Support** (Milk thistle, Dandelion root, NAC): Facilitates detoxification of estrogen and environmental toxins.

- **Minerals** (Zinc, Magnesium, Selenium): Act as co-factors in hormone production and receptor sensitivity.

- **Omega-3s & Healthy Fats**: Essential for building hormone molecules and reducing inflammation.

Nutritional support should be paired with **food-as-medicine** strategies that prioritize whole foods, blood sugar stability, and anti-inflammatory eating.

3. Lifestyle Medicine: The Foundation of Endocrine Health

Hormones do not function in a vacuum. They respond to how we **sleep, move, relate, and recover.** Lifestyle interventions are often the most potent and overlooked tools in hormone balance:

- **Stress Reduction**: Chronic stress is one of the most common causes of hormone dysregulation. Incorporating daily rituals of rest, stillness, and parasympathetic activation is non-negotiable.

- **Sleep Optimization**: Deep sleep is when the endocrine system resets. Restoring circadian rhythms through consistent bedtimes, screen hygiene, and darkened environments can rapidly shift hormone levels.

- **Movement as Medicine**: Resistance training, yoga, and rhythmic movement all have unique benefits for testosterone production, estrogen clearance, lymphatic flow, and nervous system regulation.

Clients must understand that consistency—not perfection—is the goal. Micro-shifts create macro-healing.

4. Somatic and Emotional Release:
Healing Hormonal Trauma

The endocrine system is intimately tied to the nervous system and emotional body. Trauma, especially developmental or sexual trauma, is often stored in the **reproductive organs, pelvic bowl, and fascia.** These unresolved imprints can disrupt hormonal signaling and energetic flow.

Effective somatic therapies include:

- **Somatic Experiencing (SE)** to release stored charge from the nervous system

- **Pelvic floor therapy** for women and men with reproductive tension, trauma, or pain

- **Breathwork** and **bioenergetic practices** to move stagnant energy and activate hormonal centers

- **Shamanic healing** or **energy work** to restore balance in the subtle body systems that influence hormonal health

Clients often report improved cycles, libido, and emotional stability after integrating these practices into their healing journey.

Integration is the Medicine

The most successful outcomes arise when all of these layers—biological, emotional, nutritional, spiritual—are addressed **in synergy.** Hormones are dynamic messengers; they don't just respond to what we eat or how we sleep. They respond to how we **feel, express, connect, and love.**

> "The body speaks through its hormones—our job is to learn how to listen."
> — Dr. Deilen Michelle Villegas

Hormones as Messengers of Balance

Hormones are not just biological substances—they are **the**

language of the body's inner wisdom, constantly delivering messages about safety, stress, nourishment, connection, and alignment. They are rhythmic, intelligent, and responsive to both internal perception and external conditions. When functioning optimally, they allow us to experience emotional stability, mental clarity, sexual vitality, and physical health. When dysregulated, they become **warning signals**—not of failure, but of imbalance.

Instead of suppressing symptoms with quick fixes or labeling them as disorders, we must **learn to decode the body's biochemical communication.** A missed period, low libido, sudden weight gain, mood swings, insomnia—these are not random or shameful disruptions. They are indicators that something deeper is out of sync: perhaps chronic stress, unresolved trauma, nutrient depletion, or relational disconnection.

Hormones mirror our **inner and outer environments.** For example:

- **Elevated cortisol** may reveal long-term survival mode, often stemming from unprocessed trauma, workaholism, or emotional suppression.

- **Low progesterone** might reflect a life devoid of rest, restoration, and emotional regulation.

- **Fluctuating testosterone** can signal identity struggles, burnout, or even a crisis of purpose and direction.

In this light, hormone imbalances are not problems to fix, but **portals into healing.** They ask us to listen more closely—to how we move through the world, how we nurture ourselves, and how we create space for joy, connection, and authenticity.

When clients begin to see their hormonal shifts not as betrayals but as **wisdom**, a profound transformation occurs.

They move from self-judgment to self-inquiry. From shame to sovereignty. They learn that healing is not about forcing the body into compliance, but **partnering with it**—honoring its cues and responding with compassion and alignment.

Hormonal balance is not about perfection or always feeling energized or aroused. It's about **rhythm, resilience, and relationship with self.** And as we deepen that relationship, we discover that our bodies are not broken—they are brilliantly communicating our deepest needs.

> "Your symptoms are not the problem—they are the body's solution trying to get your attention."
> — Dr. Deilen Michelle Villegas

References

Berger, A., Boggiano, M. M., & Atkinson, R. L. (2022). Neuroendocrine regulation of GABAergic activity by progesterone: Effects on mood and sleep. *Journal of Neuroendocrinology, 34*(3), e13076. https://doi.org/10.1111/jne.13076

Gore, A. C., Chappell, V. A., Fenton, S. E., Flaws, J. A., Nadal, A., Prins, G. S., ... & Zoeller, R. T. (2015). EDC-2: The Endocrine Society's Second Scientific Statement on Endocrine-Disrupting Chemicals. *Endocrine Reviews, 36*(6), E1–E150. https://doi.org/10.1210/er.2015-1010

CHAPTER 4

Postpartum Depression & Hormonal Shifts

When the Joy Turns Heavy

The postpartum period is a sacred threshold—a time of profound transformation where life is not only given to a child but also to a newly emerging mother. Yet beneath the pastel-colored images of contentment and swaddled perfection lies a **silent epidemic of suffering**. Postpartum depression (PPD) affects **1 in 7 birthing individuals**, and yet many suffer in silence, ashamed that what was supposed to be the happiest time of their life feels like an emotional collapse.

This emotional collapse is not simply "baby blues" or hormonal moodiness—it is a **neuroendocrine storm**, a **biochemical free-fall** that follows the intense hormonal elevation of pregnancy. During gestation, levels of **estrogen and progesterone rise up to 100 times their normal range** to support the growing fetus, maintain the uterine environment, and prime the brain for maternal attachment. Immediately after birth, however, those hormones **plummet within 24 to 72 hours**, leaving the brain and body scrambling for equilibrium.

This drop doesn't happen in a vacuum. **Oxytocin surges** during labor and breastfeeding, supporting bonding and maternal instinct, but without enough **dopamine and serotonin to stabilize mood and energy**, that oxytocin can turn from connection to crushing responsibility. Add in **sleep deprivation, cortisol dysregulation, nutritional depletion (especially B vitamins, magnesium, and DHA), thyroid shifts, blood sugar instability, and cultural isolation**, and you have the perfect storm for postpartum mental health collapse.

> "We don't just birth babies—we birth new versions of ourselves. But if the hormonal terrain is unstable, the self can fracture instead of integrate."
> — Dr. Deilen Michelle Villegas

Identity Reorganization: The Psychological Earthquake

PPD is not just a chemical reaction—it is an **identity crisis**. The postpartum brain undergoes structural changes that shrink the amygdala (fear center) and heighten empathy and vigilance. The mother becomes biologically wired to prioritize the infant—but at the cost of her own identity, autonomy, and sometimes, sanity.

When societal structures fail to support this transformation —when there is no community, no elder circle, no paid leave, no space for emotional honesty—**grief festers beneath the diapers and lullabies.** Many mothers grieve the loss of their former selves, their freedom, their relationships, and the fantasy of how they thought it would feel to become a parent.

And yet, they are told to smile. To bounce back. To lose the baby weight. To be grateful.

This cognitive dissonance deepens the shame spiral: *"What's wrong with me?"* becomes the haunting refrain in their minds, when in truth, the system itself is what's sick.

A Somatic and Holistic Perspective

From a **Neurosomatic Intelligence** and trauma-informed lens, we understand that the postpartum period is a **window of neuroplasticity**—a time when the nervous system is deeply open, raw, and re-patterning. This means that:

- **Old traumas may resurface** (especially those around body autonomy, abandonment, or mother wounds).

- The nervous system may enter a **freeze or dissociative state**, especially if there was birth trauma, unexpected outcomes, or surgical intervention.

- Emotional dysregulation may not be about the baby at all—but the body trying to process the spiritual and physical enormity of what just occurred.

Therapeutic interventions during this time must be **gentle, grounding, and somatic-first.** This includes:

- **Hormonal lab testing** (thyroid, estrogen, progesterone, cortisol, iron, and Vitamin D)

- **Nutrient replenishment** with whole foods, herbs, and adaptogens

- **Somatic therapies** to re-regulate the nervous system (vagal toning, breathwork, touch therapy)

- **Ritual and rest** to honor the rite of passage

- **Partner education** so that they can recognize signs of PPD and co-regulate

Cultural Gaslighting and the Need for Structural Change

Let us be clear: postpartum depression is not a personal failing —it is the result of **biological, psychological, and cultural betrayal**. We live in a society that reveres productivity over presence, performance over healing, and appearance over depth. The lack of a postpartum village, the medical system's rush to discharge, and the glamorization of "supermom" all contribute to an **epidemic of maternal burnout and isolation**.

The healing of postpartum depression is not just about rebalancing hormones—it is about **restoring dignity,** redefining identity, and reclaiming the sacredness of the mother.

Hormonal Freefall: What Happens After Birth

The postpartum period is the most abrupt and significant **hormonal shift** in the human lifecycle—greater even than puberty or menopause. Immediately following delivery, the body undergoes a biochemical crash that sets the stage for emotional, physical, and psychological recalibration. This isn't just about "baby blues." It's a **neuroendocrine upheaval**—a fragile window where the internal ecosystem is flooded with signals of both rebirth and depletion.

Estrogen and Progesterone: The Twin Pillars Collapse

During pregnancy, estrogen and progesterone reach **staggering levels**—essential to maintaining the uterine lining, supporting fetal development, and modulating immune response. Estrogen, in particular, enhances serotonin and dopamine activity, contributing to feelings of well-being, motivation, and emotional flexibility. But within **24 to 72 hours after birth**, these hormones drop by over **90%**, collapsing the chemical scaffolding that once protected mood and cognition (Bloch et al., 2003).

This sudden drop has been likened to the hormonal withdrawal of a substance detox—where the body, once accustomed to elevated levels, now struggles to function in their absence. Without adequate support, the result can be emotional fragility, mood swings, tearfulness, irritability, or complete emotional shutdown.

Oxytocin: The Bonding Hormone with Conditions

Oxytocin, often celebrated as the "love hormone," plays a pivotal role in childbirth, uterine contractions, and breastfeeding. It floods the system during skin-to-skin contact and helps foster emotional connection between mother and infant.

However, oxytocin is **highly sensitive to context**. If birth was traumatic, rushed, overly medicalized, or if the birthing person was left feeling disempowered, oxytocin release may be blunted. Similarly, **lack of skin-to-skin contact**, **breastfeeding struggles**, or **increased stress and cortisol** can inhibit this bonding hormone. Instead of feeling the rush of connection, a new parent may feel detached, numb, or even repelled—leading to increased guilt and confusion.

Cortisol: From Survival to Hypervigilance

While estrogen and progesterone crash, **cortisol—the body's stress hormone—remains elevated**. During pregnancy, cortisol gradually rises to prepare both mother and fetus for the stress of labor and delivery. In the early postpartum period, cortisol continues to surge, supporting alertness and protective instincts, but also contributing to:

- **Sleep disturbances** (even when the baby is asleep)

- **Hypervigilance** (overanalyzing baby's breathing, crying, feeding)

- **Anxiety** or **racing thoughts**

- **Startle response** and nervous system hyperactivity

If cortisol remains high without opportunities for **restorative regulation**—through sleep, nourishment, social support, and parasympathetic practices—it can lead to **adrenal burnout, mood dysregulation, and depletion of other key hormones**.

Prolactin: Nourishment and the Cost of Caregiving

Prolactin is the hormone responsible for **milk production** and **maternal caregiving behaviors**. It increases postpartum to sustain lactation and promote a nurturing, protective state.

Yet prolactin has an inverse relationship with **dopamine**, the neurotransmitter associated with motivation, desire, and pleasure. This means the longer prolactin remains elevated—especially during **night feedings, round-the-clock care, and emotional overexertion**—the more depleted dopamine may become. Over time, this can manifest as:

- **Low libido**

- **Anhedonia** (loss of pleasure or interest)

- **Fatigue and apathy**

- **Brain fog and forgetfulness**

While prolactin plays a vital role in bonding and nourishing a child, if **dopamine and oxytocin are not replenished**, the parent may begin to feel **emotionally depleted**, disconnected, or even resentful.

Key Hormonal Shifts in the Postpartum Body: A Clinical Snapshot

Hormone	Postpartum Shift	Effects on Body & Mind
Estrogen	↓ ↓ ↓	Mood instability, decreased serotonin, vaginal dryness, brain fog
Progesterone	↓ ↓ ↓	Anxiety, poor sleep, low GABA, increased PMS-like symptoms
Oxytocin	Fluctuates	Supports bonding, but is easily disrupted by stress or trauma
Cortisol	↑ ↑	Anxiety, hypervigilance,

		poor sleep, adrenal strain
Prolactin	↑	Milk production, emotional sensitivity, dopamine suppression
Dopamine & Serotonin	↓ ↓	Low motivation, anhedonia, depressive symptoms

Integrative Takeaway

Postpartum hormone shifts don't just "pass" with time—they require **intentional regulation**, replenishment, and support. Left unaddressed, this hormonal chaos can contribute to **postpartum depression, anxiety, rage, or long-term endocrine dysfunction**.

But with the right framework—**functional testing, emotional support, somatic care, and lifestyle medicine**—we can guide birthing individuals back to hormonal harmony, helping them reclaim their joy, purpose, and power.

Case Study: "Shanice's" Silent Spiral

Shanice, a 31-year-old African American first-time mother, came to counseling five months postpartum. She described feeling "disconnected from herself," overwhelmed by guilt for not enjoying motherhood the way she thought she would. Her OB-GYN had dismissed her concerns as "baby blues."

Further assessment revealed:

- Sleep deprivation averaging 3 hours per night
- High cortisol and low estrogen markers
- Isolation due to lack of partner support and culturally insensitive care

An integrative approach was applied:

- Gentle somatic therapy to support body awareness and grounding
- Nutritional support: Omega-3s, B-vitamins, magnesium
- Lactation-safe adaptogens (e.g., ashwagandha) to regulate stress
- Culturally congruent peer support groups for Black mothers

Within 8 weeks, Shanice reported reduced intrusive thoughts, improved bonding with her baby, and a more stable emotional baseline.

Psychoneuroimmunology of PPD

Postpartum depression (PPD) is not simply a hormonal imbalance or a psychological burden—it is a multidimensional condition that sits at the intersection of the nervous system, immune response, endocrine function, and lived experience. The field of **psychoneuroimmunology (PNI)** offers a powerful lens to understand how the body's communication systems can become dysregulated in the postpartum period, creating a biological environment ripe for depression, anxiety, and emotional dysregulation.

Inflammation: The Silent Amplifier of Mood Disorders

Emerging research reveals that **inflammatory cytokines**, such as interleukin-6 (IL-6), tumor necrosis factor-alpha (TNF-α), and C-reactive protein (CRP), are significantly elevated in individuals experiencing PPD (Skalkidou et al., 2009). These pro-inflammatory markers are not just byproducts of infection or physical trauma—they are **neuroactive compounds** that cross the blood-brain barrier and directly influence **neurotransmitter synthesis**, particularly serotonin, dopamine, and glutamate.

When inflammation is high:

- **Tryptophan** (a precursor to serotonin) is diverted down the kynurenine pathway, decreasing serotonin availability and increasing neurotoxic metabolites that may impair mood and cognition.

- **Dopamine production** is impaired, reducing motivation, pleasure, and emotional resilience.

- **Glutamate excitotoxicity** may increase, heightening anxiety and sleep disruption.

This inflammatory state is further intensified by **sleep deprivation**, **nutrient depletion**, **birth trauma**, and **stress**—creating a vicious cycle where the immune system fuels emotional suffering.

ACEs, Trauma, and Nervous System Priming

Another layer in this neuroimmune web is the **history of trauma**. Women and birthing individuals with a background of **adverse childhood experiences (ACEs)**, unresolved trauma, or intergenerational stress often exhibit a **sensitized HPA axis** (hypothalamic-pituitary-adrenal axis). This makes their stress response system **hyperreactive** to the immense hormonal and environmental changes of the postpartum period.

In essence, the body is already "primed" to interpret stress as threat:

- Birth, even when medically smooth, may **trigger somatic memories** of past pain or violation.

- The lack of control, bodily exposure, and medical interventions may mirror **past powerlessness**, activating the **dorsal vagal shutdown** or **sympathetic overdrive**.

- As a result, the brain may read postpartum hormonal changes as trauma, rather than transition—locking the body into a **protective survival mode** rather than a state of nurturing, bonding, and healing.

Cultural Silencing and Internalized Shame

On top of the biological storm, many new mothers face **cultural expectations of joy, gratitude, and perfection**. When their lived experience doesn't match the societal script, shame often takes root. This **shame-stress-inflammation loop** suppresses oxytocin, elevates cortisol, and stifles nervous system repair—making it nearly impossible to "just snap out of it" or "enjoy the moment."

The Clinical and Holistic Implication

Understanding the psychoneuroimmunology of PPD moves us **away from blame** and **toward biology**. It validates the lived reality of countless birthing people whose symptoms have been minimized, dismissed, or misdiagnosed. This framework also opens the door for **integrative interventions** that go beyond traditional talk therapy, including:

- **Anti-inflammatory nutritional protocols** (omega-3s, curcumin, turmeric, magnesium)

- **Nervous system regulation tools** (vagal toning, somatic therapy, trauma release)

- **Herbal adaptogens and functional medicine testing**

- **Psychoeducation for partners and families** to reduce stigma and increase co-regulation

- **Attachment-informed therapy** that addresses neurodevelopmental wounds

"PPD is not a mental weakness—it is the body's cry for restoration, integration, and safety." — Dr. Villegas

Traditional Postpartum Healing Practices Across Cultures

The postpartum period is not merely a physical recovery window—it is a sacred rite of passage. Across cultures, this transitional time is treated with reverence, ritual, and intentional support. These ancestral healing traditions acknowledge what modern medicine often overlooks: that childbirth is a profound physiological, emotional, and spiritual transformation.

Whereas Western models prioritize rapid return to "normal," rooted in productivity and independence, traditional societies see the postpartum window as an essential healing portal that shapes long-term well-being—for both mother and child.

Cuarentena (Latin America)

Cuarenta días de cuidado y contención.

Cuarentena, meaning "quarantine," refers to the **forty-day period of rest and restoration** following birth, deeply rooted in Latinx, Afro-Caribbean, and Indigenous Mesoamerican customs. During this time:

- The mother abstains from sex, housework, and heavy lifting.

- She is kept warm and nourished with **caldo de pollo** (chicken broth), **atoles**, teas, and other grounding foods.

- Elders or *parteras* (traditional midwives) offer support with **herbal teas**, **belly wrapping**, and emotional attunement.

- The focus is on **womb closure**, emotional grounding,

and **energetic restoration**.

This practice honors the womb as a sacred center and recognizes that postpartum depletion—if ignored—can lead to long-term imbalances.

Yuezi (China)

"Zuo yuezi"—Sitting the month.

In Chinese medicine, postpartum is known as the **"fourth trimester,"** where the mother is seen as energetically open and vulnerable. **Yuezi** or "sitting the month" includes:

- **No cold foods or drinks**—instead warm soups like congee, red dates, and bone broths.

- **No bathing in cold water**; instead, **herbal body washes** and warming baths.

- Wearing **thick socks and head coverings** to prevent "wind" from entering the body.

- Receiving **daily massages** and being encouraged to sleep, rest, and **bond with the baby**.

The belief is that **Qi (life force)** must be rebuilt through warmth, nourishment, and stillness. Ignoring these practices is thought to invite chronic conditions later in life, such as joint pain or mental fog.

Japa (India)

The Ayurvedic postpartum window of care.

In Ayurveda, the postpartum period is called **Sutika Kala**, and traditionally lasts 42 days. During **Japa**, the mother is treated as **"goddess in residence"** and is provided with:

- **Daily warm oil massages** (*Abhyanga*) using sesame or

medicated oils to regulate *Vata dosha* (air + ether).

- **Ghee-rich foods** and herbal soups to restore Ojas (vitality).

- **Herbal baths** with turmeric, neem, and ashwagandha to cleanse and reduce inflammation.

- Rest, chanting, prayer, and emotional support from women in the family or hired caregivers (*Japa maids*).

This time is framed not as convalescence, but as a sacred rebalancing of body and spirit.

Yoni Steaming & Sitz Baths (African, Caribbean, and Indigenous Traditions)

Womb-centered care is central in many African diasporic and Indigenous cultures. **Yoni steaming** and **herbal sitz baths** are widely used postpartum to:

- Support **perineal healing** and reduce inflammation.

- Promote **uterine cleansing** and assist with lochia release.

- Facilitate **energetic purification**—releasing trauma, grief, or spiritual residue from the birthing portal.

Herbs like **mugwort, basil, rosemary, lavender, and yarrow** are chosen based on the woman's needs and lineage-specific rituals. These practices were often passed down through oral tradition and midwifery lineage, disrupted by colonization but now being reclaimed through birthwork and ancestral healing circles.

Shared Themes Across Cultures:

Across these diverse practices, the underlying wisdom converges on key principles:

- **Warmth**: Both physical and emotional warmth —through food, environment, and connection—helps stabilize the nervous system and restore energetic boundaries.

- **Rest**: Rebuilding the body's reserves and avoiding re-entry into stress cycles or overexertion too soon.

- **Nourishment**: Food is seen not just as fuel, but as medicine—designed to rebuild blood, support lactation, and calm the nervous system.

- **Touch**: Therapeutic touch from trusted caregivers recalibrates oxytocin and promotes co-regulation.

- **Community**: The postpartum person is surrounded, not isolated. Elders, doulas, and kin provide ongoing presence, storytelling, and spiritual care.

"In traditional cultures, we do not send a woman home with a baby and a pamphlet. We send her into a sacred cocoon of care —because we know the mother is the blueprint for the next generation." — Dr. Deilen Michelle Villegas

Visual: Postpartum Hormonal Trajectory & Risk Factors

Hormone	Pre-Birth Levels	Post-Birth Drop	Mental Health Impact
Estrogen	1000x normal levels	Plummets in 3 days	Mood swings, depression
Progesterone	Elevated during pregnancy	Drops immediately	Anxiety, insomnia
Oxytocin	Rises with labor/ bonding	Variable post-birth	Impacts bonding, mood
Cortisol	High during birth	Gradual decline	Vigilance, stress sensitivity

| Prolactin | Peaks with breastfeeding | Sustained if nursing | Fatigue, emotional flattening |

Clinical Tools for Support & Recovery

Postpartum recovery requires more than symptom management—it calls for a multidimensional healing approach that addresses the **biological, emotional, neurological, and relational terrain** of the birthing individual. The following tools offer practitioners and caregivers a trauma-informed, neurobiologically sound roadmap for support.

Hormone Testing

Although the body requires time to recalibrate after birth, **comprehensive hormone testing** (once breastfeeding is established or concluded, or in acute cases of distress) can reveal critical imbalances contributing to postpartum depression, fatigue, anxiety, or brain fog.

- **DUTCH test or serum panels** may assess:

  o Estradiol, progesterone, testosterone

  o Cortisol awakening response and adrenal sufficiency

  o Thyroid function (TSH, free T3/T4, reverse T3, antibodies)

  o Nutrient co-factors like B12 and vitamin D

This data informs **individualized recovery protocols**, moving away from blanket diagnoses and toward targeted healing.

> "Testing doesn't just confirm imbalance—it gives the mother permission to trust her inner knowing."
> – Dr. Deilen Michelle Villegas

Somatic Therapy

The body remembers birth. Whether the delivery was empowering or traumatic, the **nervous system stores cellular memory**—in the pelvic floor, diaphragm, and fascia. Somatic approaches such as:

- **Somatic Experiencing (SE)**

- **TRE (Tension & Trauma Release Exercises)**

- **Craniosacral therapy**

- **Pelvic floor therapy with trauma-informed providers**

...can support nervous system discharge, increase body awareness, and rebuild the mother's connection to her own body. This is especially vital for clients who experienced emergency C-sections, obstetric violence, medical gaslighting, or sexual trauma reactivation during labor.

Mindfulness and Breathwork

Mindfulness practices reconnect the postpartum body to presence—essential when the mind is foggy, hypervigilant, or emotionally overwhelmed. **Simple breathwork protocols** (such as 4-7-8 breathing or alternate nostril breathing) help regulate:

- **Cortisol and adrenaline** spikes from sleep deprivation

- **Anxiety loops** around safety or performance

- **Heart rate variability (HRV)** to support parasympathetic tone

- **Oxytocin production**, especially when combined with skin-to-skin contact or touch-based rituals

Guided meditations focused on **self-compassion**, **mother archetype reintegration**, and **identity transformation** can help anchor the emotional rebirth occurring alongside physical recovery.

Nutrition and Supplementation

Nutritional deficiencies are common postpartum due to blood loss, nutrient diversion to breastmilk, and chronic stress. Key areas of focus include:

- **Iron**: Prevents anemia, supports energy and cognition

- **Vitamin D**: Modulates immunity, mood, and inflammation

- **B12 and folate**: Essential for neurochemical synthesis and fatigue prevention

- **DHA and omega-3s**: Crucial for brain health and hormone production

- **Adaptogens**: Ashwagandha, reishi, shatavari, and holy basil can regulate cortisol and support thyroid/adrenal restoration (always review lactation safety)

Encouraging warm, grounding, nutrient-dense foods—**bone broths, root vegetables, warming spices, and healthy fats**—honors traditional postpartum principles and supports biochemical healing.

Partner and Family Education

Support is not just maternal—it's **relational and systemic**. Educating partners, parents, and family members on:

- The **emotional and hormonal terrain** of postpartum

- Signs of PPD or trauma

- The importance of **nonjudgmental listening**

- **Shared caregiving models**

- How to increase oxytocin through safe touch, presence, and attunement

...can reduce resentment, increase bonding, and decrease isolation. When loved ones understand that the postpartum person is navigating **neurochemical recalibration**, not "moodiness," they become co-healers, not critics.

"Postpartum healing is not a solo journey. It requires a village rooted in science, compassion, and ancestral wisdom." — Dr. Deilen Michelle Villegas

Postpartum Plan for Moms and Partners

Bringing new life into the world changes everything—body, brain, identity, and relationships. The postpartum period is not a recovery from weakness, but a **regeneration of power**. It requires conscious support, deep listening, and rituals that protect both the sacred bond with the child and the health of the birthing person.

This plan offers a **practical, trauma-informed, and culturally respectful** framework for both mothers and their partners to navigate the early postpartum window with intention.

For Mothers: Replenish, Regulate, Receive

This is not a time to "bounce back"—this is your season to root in, to rebuild, and to receive.

Prioritize Restorative Sleep (When Possible)

- Short naps throughout the day are not lazy—they're medicine.

- Sleep hygiene may include blackout curtains, magnesium, or gentle sleep teas.

- If baby is safe and fed, it's okay to let the dishes wait.

Nourish with Warming, Grounding Foods

- Bone broths, root vegetables, oatmeal, stews, and herbal infusions support digestion and womb recovery.

- Focus on **iron-rich foods**, **healthy fats**, and **hydration with electrolytes** to replenish blood and energy.

- Minimize cold/raw foods which may disrupt digestive fire in some traditions.

Delegate & Protect Your Energy

- Ask for (or receive) help with laundry, meals, errands, or infant care.

- Limit visitors—*your healing comes first.*

- Say no with grace and without guilt.

Gentle Movement to Support Circulation and Mood

- Breathwork calms the nervous system and supports hormonal recalibration.

- Walking in nature, stretching, or pelvic floor exercises can gently reconnect body and spirit.

- Somatic practices help release trauma stored during labor or from earlier life experiences.

Skin-to-Skin & Oxytocin Rituals

- Hold baby to your chest as often as possible, especially after feedings.

- Use music, scent, and voice to create a calming bonding environment.

- Let oxytocin be your guiding hormone—not cortisol.

  "You are not just recovering from birth—you are becoming. Rest is sacred. Nourishment is non-negotiable."

For Partners: Anchor, Attune, Advocate

Support is more than logistics—it's **emotional fluency, shared responsibility**, and **presence without pressure**.

Validate Emotions Without Fixing

- "It's okay to feel that way" can be more powerful than advice.

- Postpartum feelings may range from joy to rage to grief. Hold them all with compassion.

Share the Load

- Night feeds, diaper changes, meal prep, or baby-wearing allow the mother to rest and recover.

- Ask, "What would feel most supportive today?"—then *do it.*

Touch with Intention, Not Expectation

- Light massage, back rubs, or holding her hand during tears speaks volumes.

- Postpartum touch should be safe, slow, and consent-based—especially if trauma was involved in birth.

Watch for Signs of Distress, Not Just Symptoms

- Notice changes in mood, sleep, or bonding. Is she withdrawing, overwhelmed, or persistently sad?

- Encourage help without shame. Say: *"You're not broken—you're recalibrating. Let's reach out together."*

Protect Sacred Space

- Limit screens and overstimulation. Create "tech-free" zones.

- Light a candle, play calming music, and create rituals for presence: baby baths, slow dinners, storytime.

  "Presence is protection. When partners regulate their nervous systems, they become a sanctuary—not a stressor."

Joint Healing Practices

- **Co-regulation**: Practice breathwork or meditation together.

- **Intimacy Reset**: Redefine closeness as cuddling, conversation, shared silence—not just sex.

- **Gratitude Rituals**: Share one thing you're grateful for about each other each night.

- **Weekly Check-Ins**: Use nonviolent communication to express needs, boundaries, and appreciations.

"Postpartum care is not just about the baby's health—it is a rite of passage for the parent, and we must treat it as such." — Dr. Deilen Michelle Villegas

Rewriting the Narrative

The postpartum window is not just a recovery period—it is a **rite of passage**, a neurological, emotional, and spiritual reorganization of identity. Yet in modern Western culture, this sacred transformation is too often framed in sterile, clinical terms or overlooked entirely. We medicalize birth through interventions, checklists, and hospital protocols—but we neglect the **mind-body-spirit terrain** that unfolds afterward. In doing so, we abandon mothers, birthing people, and families in a landscape of invisible wounds.

Postpartum depression (PPD) is not just a mental health diagnosis—it is a **biopsychosocial experience** rooted in hormonal withdrawal, identity disorientation, inflammatory markers, unmet emotional needs, and systemic lack of care. When we treat it solely with medication or overlook it entirely, we risk pathologizing what is often a **natural call for reconnection, nourishment, and integration.**

Rewriting this narrative means **de-shaming the experience**, expanding our definitions of postpartum wellness, and validating the entire spectrum of emotions that can surface. It means normalizing the grief that can coexist with joy, the rage that can arise beside love, and the fear that walks hand-in-hand with awe. These are not signs of dysfunction—they are signs of **awakening in a nervous system seeking equilibrium** after profound transformation.

In holistic and trauma-informed care models, we ask:

- **What does this parent need to feel safe again in their body?**

- **Where did their support systems fail them—medically, emotionally, spiritually?**

- **What ancestral wisdom can we return to that honors this transition, rather than rushing through it?**

- **How can we speak to the nervous system through food, touch, words, and stillness—not just prescriptions and protocols?**

When we honor postpartum as a **neurochemical unfolding**, a **somatic recalibration**, and a **spiritual rebirth**, we create the conditions for true healing—not just symptom management.

"Healing begins when we stop treating postpartum depression as a problem to fix—and begin to see it as a message from the soul asking to be held, seen, and re-integrated." — Dr. Deilen Michelle Villegas

References

Bloch, M., Schmidt, P. J., Danaceau, M., Murphy, J., Nieman, L., & Rubinow, D. R. (2003). Effects of gonadal steroids in women with a history of postpartum depression. *American Journal of Psychiatry, 160*(4), 908-915. https://doi.org/10.1176/appi.ajp.160.4.908

Skalkidou, A., Sylvén, S. M., Papadopoulos, F. C., Olovsson, M., Larsson, A., & Sundström Poromaa, I. (2009). Risk of postpartum depression in association with serum leptin and interleukin-6 levels at delivery: A nested case–control study within the UPPSAT cohort. *Psychoneuroendocrinology, 34*(9), 1329-1337. https://doi.org/10.1016/j.psyneuen.2009.03.004

CHAPTER 5

Medication & Post-SSRI Sexual Dysfunction

When Relief Comes at a Cost

Selective serotonin reuptake inhibitors (SSRIs) have revolutionized the treatment of depression and anxiety, including postpartum depression, trauma-related disorders, and generalized anxiety. For many, they offer a lifeline—relief from despair, panic, or emotional numbness. But too often, the long-term effects on **sexual function, hormonal health, and emotional intimacy** are overlooked in the pursuit of emotional stabilization.

One of the most underreported and poorly understood consequences is **Post-SSRI Sexual Dysfunction (PSSD)**—a condition in which individuals experience long-term sexual side effects even after discontinuing the medication. These effects can include diminished libido, anorgasmia (inability to reach orgasm), genital numbness, erectile dysfunction, delayed ejaculation, and emotional blunting. In many cases, these symptoms persist for months or even years after the drug has been stopped, impacting **self-esteem, body image, relationships, and mental health.**

> "Healing the mind should never come at the cost of silencing the body's capacity for pleasure." — Dr. Deilen Michelle Villegas

SSRIs work by increasing serotonin in the brain, a neurotransmitter associated with mood regulation. However, serotonin also **inhibits dopamine and oxytocin pathways** —key players in sexual arousal, pleasure, bonding, and motivation. Over time, elevated serotonin levels can **dampen**

dopaminergic sensitivity, blunt emotional intensity, and desensitize genital arousal pathways.

Additionally, SSRIs may suppress **testosterone production**, alter thyroid function, and disrupt cortisol rhythms—contributing to fatigue, brain fog, weight gain, and further sexual decline. For birthing individuals in the postpartum period or clients already struggling with hormonal imbalances, the cumulative effect can be emotionally devastating.

The Emotional Fallout of PSSD

Sexual dysfunction is not just a physical issue—it impacts the nervous system, sense of self, and relational safety. Clients may report feeling "disconnected from their body," "numb during intimacy," or as though "the spark is gone." In partnerships, this can lead to **resentment, performance anxiety, self-withdrawal, or shame.** Tragically, many individuals are dismissed when they bring up these concerns, being told it's "all in their head" or a necessary trade-off for mental wellness.

But pleasure is not a luxury—it is a core component of **nervous system regulation, hormonal vitality, and identity integration**. To rob someone of their embodied pleasure while treating their depression is to fragment the healing process.

Clinical Support Strategies for PSSD

A trauma-informed and integrative approach to supporting post-SSRI sexual dysfunction includes:

- **Functional Testing**: Assess neurotransmitter imbalances, testosterone/cortisol levels, and nutrient depletions (e.g., B6, zinc, magnesium).

- **Amino Acid Therapy**: Support dopamine and oxytocin production with L-tyrosine, phenylalanine, mucuna pruriens, or SAMe under supervision.

- **Pelvic-Somatic Therapy**: Reconnect clients to sensation through body-based healing practices, breathwork, yoni/lingam mapping, and mindful self-touch.

- **Adaptogenic Herbs**: Use herbs like maca, ashwagandha, or tribulus to support hormonal vitality and libido.

- **Mindfulness & Erotic Reclamation**: Teach clients how to re-engage with their sensual self using erotic blueprints, mirror work, and non-goal-based touch.

- **Couples Work**: Rebuild emotional and physical safety in relationships through communication exercises, oxytocin rituals, and education on neurochemical recovery.

Rethinking the Standard of Care

Mental health care must evolve to include **sexual well-being as a core pillar** of healing—not an optional afterthought. Clients deserve full transparency when prescribed medication and ongoing support if side effects compromise their quality of life.

In trauma-informed practice, we ask not only *"What symptoms are we treating?"* but also *"What parts of this client are we silencing in the process?"*

"To heal is not only to feel less pain—but to feel more pleasure, more connection, more aliveness. We must never forget this truth in our clinical approach." — Dr. Deilen Michelle Villegas

The Mechanism of SSRIs

Selective serotonin reuptake inhibitors (SSRIs) are widely

prescribed for conditions such as depression, anxiety, obsessive-compulsive disorder (OCD), and postpartum depression. Their efficacy stems from their ability to **increase serotonin levels** in the synaptic cleft by preventing its reabsorption (reuptake) into the presynaptic neuron. This elevated serotonin is often associated with improved mood, reduced rumination, and enhanced emotional resilience.

However, the body operates on a **delicate neurochemical ecosystem**, where enhancing one neurotransmitter may suppress another. This is especially true with SSRIs, which—while elevating serotonin—**simultaneously inhibit dopamine**, norepinephrine, and even **suppress nitric oxide synthesis**, all of which are crucial for sexual arousal, desire, and orgasmic release.

> "Serotonin soothes the mind—but too much can sedate the body's natural vitality and drive." — Dr. Deilen Michelle Villegas

How SSRIs Affect Sexual Function:

- **Dopamine Suppression**: Dopamine is responsible for motivation, pleasure, and reward. It plays a central role in sexual anticipation, initiation, and climax. When serotonin rises too high, it inhibits dopamine transmission, leading to low libido, reduced erotic imagination, and difficulty reaching orgasm.

- **Nitric Oxide Inhibition**: Nitric oxide is essential for blood flow to the genitals. It supports erectile function in men and engorgement and lubrication in women. SSRIs have been shown to reduce nitric oxide synthase activity, impairing arousal at a vascular level (Clayton et al., 2006).

- **Oxytocin Disruption**: Serotonin modulates oxytocin

release, which governs feelings of bonding and emotional intimacy. Chronic SSRI use can blunt this hormonal response, leading to emotional detachment or decreased romantic bonding—even in previously secure relationships.

- **Blunted Emotional Resonance**: Emotional flattening or "blunting" is a common complaint among long-term SSRI users. Clients report feeling like they're "watching life through a window"—present but not emotionally engaged, especially in areas involving love, grief, or sexual passion.

Commonly Affected Areas of Sexual and Emotional Health:

- **Libido and Sexual Desire**: A reduced interest in initiating or responding to sexual cues.

- **Arousal Difficulties**: Trouble achieving erection, lubrication, or psychological arousal.

- **Anorgasmia or Delayed Orgasm**: Inability to climax, or a feeling that climax is muted or emotionally unfulfilling.

- **Emotional Disconnection**: Difficulty feeling romantic attachment, even in loving partnerships.

- **Reduced Genital Sensation**: Clients may describe their genitals as "numb," "dead," or "distant," contributing to shame and confusion.

These effects are not just temporary annoyances—they can deeply impact self-esteem, sexual identity, and relational harmony.

Post-SSRI Sexual Dysfunction (PSSD): The Lingering Shadow

While many individuals regain their sexual function after

tapering off SSRIs, a growing number of cases reveal **persistent dysfunction lasting months or years after cessation**—a phenomenon now recognized as **Post-SSRI Sexual Dysfunction (PSSD)**. The exact mechanism is not fully understood, but hypotheses include:

- **Epigenetic alterations** in serotonin and dopamine receptor sensitivity

- **Long-term dysregulation** of nitric oxide pathways

- **Neurological desensitization** of erogenous zones and genital sensory receptors

- **Persistent emotional blunting** due to altered limbic system processing

PSSD is not yet widely acknowledged by many providers, leading to gaslighting, dismissal, or misdiagnosis as psychological resistance rather than a legitimate neurochemical disorder. However, ongoing research and patient advocacy are pushing for recognition and support (Healy et al., 2018).

"When we flatten pleasure in the name of control, we also flatten identity, vitality, and connection. True healing honors the whole experience of being alive." — Dr. Deilen Michelle Villegas

What is Post-SSRI Sexual Dysfunction (PSSD)?

Post-SSRI Sexual Dysfunction (PSSD) is a **persistent, often debilitating condition** marked by sexual and emotional numbness that continues well after the discontinuation of selective serotonin reuptake inhibitors (SSRIs). Though still under-recognized in mainstream psychiatry, the growing body of clinical reports, research data, and patient testimonies point to PSSD as a **legitimate neurobiological and psychosexual**

disorder.

Unlike temporary side effects that resolve within weeks of stopping medication, PSSD can last **months or even years**, with symptoms showing **no correlation** to pre-existing mental health status, hormone levels, or ongoing psychiatric need. Many clients report feeling abandoned or dismissed by medical professionals, who attribute their distress to "anxiety," "depression," or "psychosomatic fixation." However, the reality is often rooted in **deep neurochemical dysregulation**.

Core Symptoms of PSSD Include:

- **Genital Numbness:** Loss of physical sensation, often described as "dead," "rubbery," or "disconnected."

- **Anorgasmia:** Inability to achieve orgasm, or orgasm that feels mechanical and emotionally flat.

- **Decreased Libido:** Lack of spontaneous desire, erotic thought, or interest in intimacy.

- **Arousal Dysfunction:** Difficulty becoming physically aroused (erection/lubrication), despite psychological willingness.

- **Emotional Numbing:** A reduction in the capacity to feel romantic love, attachment, or emotional highs.

- **Cognitive Detachment:** Feelings of depersonalization, derealization, or blunted response to beauty, music, or nature.

These symptoms are especially **distressing to young people**, many of whom were prescribed SSRIs in their teens or early twenties—during key windows of sexual and identity development.

Emerging Mechanisms and Theories Behind PSSD

While the exact pathophysiology of PSSD remains unclear, several compelling mechanisms are being explored:

- **Serotonin Receptor Desensitization:** Chronic serotonin elevation may downregulate 5-HT1A and 5-HT2A receptors, critical for dopamine release and nitric oxide synthesis—both of which are essential for arousal and pleasure.

- **Epigenetic Changes:** Prolonged SSRI use may alter gene expression involved in neuroplasticity, sensory processing, and hormonal regulation (Ben-Sheetrit et al., 2014).

- **Nitric Oxide Pathway Disruption:** SSRIs inhibit nitric oxide synthase, which plays a crucial role in vasodilation and genital blood flow. Long-term suppression may damage this system's responsiveness.

- **Dopaminergic Downregulation:** Excess serotonin suppresses dopamine, the neurotransmitter of motivation, pleasure, and reward. Over time, this can flatten erotic imagination and motivation for connection.

- **Pelvic Nerve Inhibition:** Some researchers theorize that SSRIs may alter autonomic nervous system tone in ways that desensitize pudendal and pelvic nerve communication.

Importantly, **these mechanisms often function in combination**, creating a multifaceted pattern of dysfunction that is not purely hormonal or psychological.

Case Study: Noah's Numbness

Client Background:

- **Name:** Noah (pseudonym)

- **Age:** 27

- **SSRI History:** Prescribed fluoxetine at age 21 for generalized anxiety disorder; remained on the medication for three years.

- **Discontinuation:** Tapered off under medical supervision over 18 months.

Presenting Concerns:
After full discontinuation, Noah experienced:

- Loss of morning erections and spontaneous arousal

- Genital numbness despite physical stimulation

- Difficulty forming new romantic attachments

- Shame and self-doubt, fearing he was "broken" or "no longer a man"

Initial labs showed **testosterone and thyroid hormones within normal ranges**, ruling out basic endocrine dysfunction. A deeper evaluation revealed trauma around performance failure, grief around past relationships, and a history of early attachment disruption—all layered beneath the neurochemical disruptions.

Integrative Recovery Plan:

Noah's treatment focused on **neuroregeneration, emotional integration, and somatic reconnection**. His protocol included:

- **L-arginine + Ginseng**: Amino acid support to enhance **nitric oxide synthesis** and penile blood flow.

- **Mucuna Pruriens**: A dopaminergic adaptogen to support mood, libido, and reward system activation.

- **Acupuncture + Pelvic Floor Therapy**: To stimulate blood flow and restore vagal/pudendal nerve balance.

- **Somatic Therapy**: To access blocked emotional states and rebuild mind-body intimacy.

- **Sensate Focus Exercises**: Non-goal-oriented touch and breath practices to reawaken sensual pathways.

Outcome:

After **six months**, Noah reported:

- The return of spontaneous arousal

- Improved tactile sensitivity

- The ability to orgasm again with emotional connection

- A growing sense of self-trust and embodied masculinity

"For the first time in years, I felt like my body belonged to me again." — Noah

Healing is Possible

PSSD is not a sentence—it is a **call for integrative recovery**. While there is no standardized medical cure yet, many clients find improvement with **patient, multi-modal care**. Recovery includes not just treating neurochemical imbalance, but also restoring a sense of **agency, hope, and embodied aliveness**.

Medication, Hormones & Libido

While SSRIs are primarily designed to elevate mood by increasing serotonin availability, their impact on the **neuroendocrine system**—especially the **hypothalamic-pituitary-gonadal (HPG) axis**—is often underappreciated. The HPG axis is a key regulator of reproductive and sexual health, influencing everything from libido and fertility to mood and body composition. When SSRIs interfere with this delicate feedback loop, the consequences ripple far beyond the bedroom.

Key Hormonal Disruptions Triggered by SSRIs:

Reduced Testosterone Levels (in all sexes)

- SSRIs may **inhibit the release of gonadotropin-releasing hormone (GnRH)** from the hypothalamus, which in turn suppresses luteinizing hormone (LH) and follicle-stimulating hormone (FSH) from the pituitary gland.

- This downstream suppression leads to **lower production of testosterone** in the testes (in men) and ovaries/adrenal glands (in women).

- The result? Reduced libido, fatigue, muscle loss, emotional flatness, and decreased assertiveness—all hallmarks of **androgen deficiency.**

Suppressed Luteinizing Hormone (LH) and FSH

- These hormones are critical for ovulation in women and spermatogenesis in men.

- SSRI interference can result in **anovulatory cycles, irregular periods,** and **fertility challenges** in women—even those with otherwise normal hormone levels.

- In men, lowered LH/FSH levels can contribute to **low sperm count** and decreased reproductive viability, particularly when SSRIs are taken long-term.

Interference with Estrogen and Progesterone Balance

- Serotonin has reciprocal regulatory relationships with both estrogen and progesterone.

- Disruption of these hormones can lead to:

    o Menstrual irregularity or amenorrhea

    o Exacerbation of PMS or PMDD

    o Mood instability and **heightened emotional reactivity**

    o Disconnection from feminine energy and sensual self-image

- In transgender and nonbinary individuals on hormone replacement therapy (HRT), SSRIs may **blunt the intended effects** of exogenous hormones, complicating emotional and sexual wellness goals.

The Ripple Effect: Emotional, Physical, and Relational Fallout

This **hormonal disruption does not exist in a vacuum**—it often amplifies the very symptoms for which medication was originally prescribed:

- **Mood dysregulation:** Lowered testosterone and progesterone reduce natural buffering against stress and irritability.

- **Fatigue and low motivation:** A suppressed hormonal cascade means less cellular energy, poorer mitochondrial function, and reduced resilience.

- **Body image concerns:** Hormonal shifts may lead to weight gain (especially around the midsection), water retention, and reduced muscle tone—triggering shame and discomfort in one's own body.

- **Relational distress:** Reduced libido and emotional numbing impair intimacy, communication, and mutual fulfillment in partnerships.

It becomes a **cycle of substitution**, where one kind of suffering is exchanged for another—alleviating anxiety but numbing pleasure, suppressing intrusive thoughts but also dulling vitality.

Clinical Takeaway:

True healing must consider **both symptom relief and long-term hormonal integrity**. Clients on SSRIs who present with libido loss, emotional flattening, or hormonal irregularity deserve:

- Validation of their lived experience

- Holistic education on the medication's full-body impact

- Tools to co-regulate mood and chemistry without sacrificing sensuality or identity

  "Medications may treat symptoms—but restoring connection to pleasure, presence, and power requires a more integrative path." — Dr. Villegas

Visual: SSRI Impact on Sexual Health

Domain	Impact of SSRI Use	Possible Lasting Effect (PSSD)
Libido	Decreased interest in sex	Persistent low desire
Arousal	Erectile dysfunction, vaginal dryness	Genital numbness
Orgasm	Delayed or absent orgasm	Anorgasmia
Emotion	Emotional blunting, decreased attachment	Romantic disconnection
Hormones	Suppression of testosterone, LH, estrogen	Endocrine dysregulation

Clinical Alternatives & Holistic Strategies: Reclaiming Sexual Vitality After SSRIs

Addressing SSRI-induced sexual dysfunction requires a **multifaceted, trauma-informed, and integrative** approach that honors both the neurochemical and emotional landscapes of the client. When clients report libido loss, genital numbness, emotional flatness, or difficulty connecting intimately, the goal isn't just to restore sexual function—it's to **reignite vitality, presence, and embodied joy**.

Tapering Protocols Under Medical Supervision

The first step for many clients may be to **gradually taper off SSRIs**, but this must always be done **in collaboration with a prescribing provider**. Abrupt withdrawal can result in serotonin discontinuation syndrome and emotional destabilization. A trauma-informed, body-aware tapering protocol includes:

- **Functional lab testing** (e.g., DUTCH, neurotransmitter panels)

- **Supportive therapies** like neurofeedback, EMDR, or somatic experiencing

- Gradual substitution with **nervous system tonics and mood-regulating adaptogens**

> "We don't rush the body out of survival—we guide it back into safety."

Adaptogens to Regulate the HPA Axis

Chronic SSRI use often dysregulates the **hypothalamic-pituitary-adrenal (HPA) axis**, flattening the body's stress response and hormonal flexibility. Adaptogens are plant allies that help **restore homeostasis**, increase resilience, and improve energy.

Key options include:

- **Rhodiola Rosea**: Enhances focus, motivation, and stamina while supporting dopaminergic tone.

- **Holy Basil (Tulsi)**: Calms cortisol spikes, soothes anxiety, and gently uplifts mood.

- **Ashwagandha**: Supports thyroid and testosterone production, reduces irritability, and promotes restful sleep.

These herbs work best when **paired with lifestyle changes** that support circadian health, such as consistent sleep, hydration, and reduced screen time before bed.

Dopamine Restoration Through Lifestyle Medicine

Because SSRIs blunt dopamine and pleasure pathways, restoring dopaminergic balance is crucial. Dopamine is the **"desire molecule"**—involved in motivation, reward, and sexual drive.

Holistic dopamine-boosting strategies include:

- **Nutrition**: Tyrosine-rich foods (eggs, avocados, chicken, beets) support dopamine synthesis.

- **Sunlight**: Daily light exposure boosts serotonin and dopamine through retinal activation.

- **Movement**: Cardiovascular and resistance training both upregulate dopamine and testosterone.

- **Supplementation**: Mucuna pruriens (L-dopa), L-tyrosine, vitamin B6, and magnesium.

Restoring dopamine isn't about chasing euphoria—it's about **reclaiming agency, momentum, and joy**.

Herbal Allies for Libido & Hormonal Vitality

Ancient traditions have long honored certain herbs as aphrodisiacs—not because they override the body, but because they **awaken it**. These botanical allies work through hormonal, circulatory, and energetic pathways:

- **Maca Root**: Balances estrogen/testosterone, supports adrenal health, and boosts desire

- **Tribulus Terrestris**: Enhances androgen sensitivity and improves erectile function

- **Shatavari**: Nourishes female reproductive health,

especially in those recovering from burnout or low progesterone

- **Horny Goat Weed (Epimedium)**: Supports nitric oxide production and libido, especially in men

These herbs should be used **intentionally and respectfully**, considering dosage, energetics, and potential interactions.

Sex Therapy & Somatic Reconnection

Medication may dull sensation—but the body's capacity for pleasure is **never lost, only dormant**. Through mindful, embodied reconnection, clients can restore intimacy without pressure or performance anxiety.

Clinical Tools:

- **Sensate Focus**: A touch-based practice that rebuilds intimacy through non-goal-oriented connection

- **Breathwork & Sounding**: Reignite sensual flow and emotional release

- **Erotic Blueprint Exploration**: Helps clients understand their unique arousal language

- **Mirror Work & Embodiment Exercises**: Reclaim confidence, presence, and sensual identity

In couples' work, shifting focus from intercourse to **emotional safety, consent, and play** often opens the door to deeper intimacy and pleasure.

"Sexuality is not a luxury—it's a vital sign of aliveness. When we honor desire, we honor life force itself." — Dr. Deilen Michelle Villegas

Informed Healing and Sexual Sovereignty

While SSRIs can be life-saving interventions for depression, anxiety, and trauma-related disorders, **they are not without consequence**—particularly when it comes to the realms of pleasure, connection, and sexual identity. For too long, the **sexual side effects of psychotropic medications** have been downplayed, dismissed, or ignored in clinical conversations. This omission not only erodes trust in the therapeutic process but also perpetuates the silent suffering of countless individuals.

Informed healing begins with **transparent dialogue**. Clients have the right to understand how a prescribed medication may influence not just their symptoms, but their relationships, self-image, and sensuality. Sexuality is not an optional or fringe concern—it is a central expression of **vitality, relational intimacy, hormonal health, and personal power**. When this is muted, numbed, or chemically disrupted, it can create secondary wounds that compound mental distress.

We must move beyond the binary framing of "mental health vs. sexual health" and recognize that **true healing must include both**. Clinicians must:

- Routinely assess **sexual function and satisfaction** as part of mental health evaluations

- Create space for **shame-free conversations** around libido, arousal, and emotional connection

- Offer **integrative, body-based alternatives and adjunctive support** for those exploring medication tapering or recovery

- Advocate for **sexual agency** as a fundamental aspect of trauma-informed care

Sexual sovereignty is the **reclamation of one's pleasure, body,**

boundaries, and choice. It means no longer outsourcing your experience of intimacy to a pill bottle or to someone else's expectations. It means honoring the truth of your body, even when that truth challenges clinical norms.

> "Informed consent is not just about listing side effects—it's about empowering clients to choose healing that honors their wholeness."

As practitioners, we are called not only to manage symptoms but to guide people back to themselves—back to their **sensation, spark, sacredness, and sovereignty**.

References

Ben-Sheetrit, J., Aizenberg, D., Kaplan, M. J., & Weizman, A. (2014). Post-SSRI sexual dysfunction: Clinical characterization and preliminary assessment. *International Journal of Psychiatry in Clinical Practice, 18*(3), 204–211. https://doi.org/10.3109/13651501.2014.902765

Clayton, A. H., Pradko, J. F., Croft, H. A., Montano, C. B., Leadbetter, R. A., & Bolden-Watson, C. (2006). Prevalence of sexual dysfunction among newer antidepressants. *Journal of Clinical Psychiatry, 67*(5), 713–716. https://doi.org/10.4088/JCP.v67n0501

CHAPTER 6

Infertility & Hidden Root Causes

The Unseen Battle for Conception

Infertility is often misunderstood—not just by society, but even within conventional medicine. Too frequently, the diagnosis is approached with a narrow focus on reproductive organs, ovulation cycles, or sperm count. But the **inability to conceive is rarely just about the uterus or the testes**. It is the body's alarm system signaling a deeper disruption—a systemic cry for balance and restoration.

Behind the scenes of every fertility struggle are **layers of hidden root causes**—often missed in surface-level evaluations. These include hormonal imbalances, metabolic dysfunctions, nutrient depletion, toxic overload, trauma imprints, and emotional distress. Infertility is not simply a medical obstacle; it is **a physiological puzzle woven with the threads of mind, body, and spirit**.

Hormonal Chaos: The Endocrine Web

The endocrine system is delicate, and small disruptions can lead to large consequences. When **cortisol (stress hormone)** is chronically elevated, it competes with progesterone, causing irregular cycles or anovulation. **Thyroid imbalances**, especially undiagnosed hypothyroidism or Hashimoto's, can impair implantation and disrupt pregnancy maintenance. **Insulin resistance** and androgen dominance in PCOS are other culprits that sabotage ovulatory function.

> Fertility isn't about isolated hormone levels—it's about **orchestration**, rhythm, and communication across the endocrine symphony.

The Hidden Players: Homocysteine, Inflammation, and Methylation

Elevated **homocysteine**, a byproduct of impaired methylation, has been linked to **poor egg quality, recurrent miscarriage, and preeclampsia**. Often, this elevation is driven by genetic variations (e.g., MTHFR mutations) or nutrient deficiencies in B12, B6, and folate. Addressing these biochemical imbalances not only improves fertility but enhances whole-body vitality.

Systemic inflammation—from chronic infections, gut dysbiosis, or autoimmune activity—creates a hostile internal environment for conception. An inflamed womb cannot welcome life. Healing must start by calming the body's inflammatory load through diet, detox, and nervous system regulation.

Environmental and Epigenetic Disruptors

Modern life bombards us with **endocrine-disrupting chemicals (EDCs)**—xenoestrogens in plastics, pesticides, fragrances, and processed foods. These compounds mimic natural hormones, causing estrogen dominance, low testosterone, or progesterone suppression. Over time, they distort reproductive signaling and deplete the body's ability to detox.

Heavy metals (like mercury, lead, and cadmium) also impair mitochondrial function, damage reproductive organs, and disrupt egg and sperm quality. Detoxification protocols must be safe, supervised, and integrated with nutritional repletion and nervous system support.

Trauma, Shame, and the Emotional Womb

Many people trying to conceive are carrying **unresolved trauma in the pelvic space**—whether from sexual abuse, medical trauma, ancestral grief, or internalized shame. This trauma can lead to energetic blockages, tension in the fascia and pelvic floor, or even subconscious resistance to conception.

Somatic therapies, breathwork, trauma-informed bodywork, and womb healing practices can help release these emotional imprints. When the body feels safe, soft, and sovereign, it becomes more receptive to life.

> "You cannot force life to grow in a place that feels unsafe. Healing the emotional terrain is as critical as balancing the hormonal one." --Dr. Deilen Michelle Villegas

Case Insight: Mila's Journey

Mila, a 36-year-old Latina woman, came to my clinic after three years of failed fertility treatments. Her labs were "normal," yet she experienced irregular cycles, chronic bloating, fatigue, and anxiety. Upon deeper investigation, we found:

- Elevated homocysteine

- Mold exposure in her home

- Childhood sexual trauma and a deeply internalized sense of unworthiness

- A history of over-exercising and under-eating

Her healing plan included:

- Methylation support (methylated B12, folate, magnesium)

- Mold detox protocol

- Somatic healing and guided womb meditations

- Shifting to a fertility-nourishing diet with warming, nutrient-rich foods

- Partner intimacy sessions to rebuild safety and sensual connection

Within nine months, Mila conceived naturally. More than the pregnancy itself, what she reclaimed was her power, her voice, and her trust in her body.

Reframing Infertility as Insight

Infertility is not a dead end. It is a mirror, reflecting areas of the body that require deeper nourishment, care, and curiosity. By moving beyond reductionist medicine and embracing an integrative, trauma-informed, and holistic approach, we begin to **transform infertility from pathology into possibility**.

> "Infertility is not the end of the story—it's an invitation to listen to what the body has been trying to say all along." — Dr. Deilen Michelle Villegas

The Rise of Infertility in Modern Society

Infertility is no longer a rare or isolated issue—it is a **growing public health concern**, reflective of larger systemic imbalances in modern life. According to the World Health Organization, roughly **1 in 6 couples** globally face infertility challenges. Yet even with its increasing prevalence, conversations around infertility remain overly simplified, often placing the burden on the uterus, ovaries, or age—neglecting the vast ecosystem of physiological, environmental, and emotional factors that affect reproductive health.

In reality, **infertility is a symptom of a larger disconnect**— between humans and their bodies, between science and the soul, and between modern living and the natural rhythms of the body.

Infertility Is Not Just a "Woman's Issue"

Despite pervasive narratives, **infertility is equally likely to originate from male factors**, including poor sperm quality, motility issues, hormonal dysregulation, or testicular inflammation. And yet, the diagnostic process often disproportionately focuses on female reproductive organs. A truly integrative, functional approach must explore the **full-body, whole-person perspective**—regardless of sex or gender identity.

Lesser-Known Physiological Contributors to Infertility

These root contributors often go undetected in conventional fertility assessments but are vital to consider when taking a holistic view.

Elevated Homocysteine Levels

Homocysteine is a sulfur-containing amino acid that, when elevated, becomes a silent saboteur of fertility. It creates systemic **inflammation**, damages vascular linings, and impairs implantation.

- Linked to: **recurrent miscarriage, poor egg quality, placental dysfunction**

- Root causes: **MTHFR mutations**, poor methylation, deficiencies in **B6, B12, folate**

- Clinical insight: Women with high homocysteine often present with fatigue, anxiety, or poor detox capacity, yet rarely are they screened unless cardiovascular issues arise.

Scar Tissue and Pelvic Adhesions

Often the result of:

- **Past surgeries** (e.g., C-section, appendectomy)

- **Endometriosis** or **Pelvic Inflammatory Disease (PID)**

- **Sexually transmitted infections**

Scar tissue creates physical barriers:

- **Obstructing fallopian tubes**

- **Distorting uterine position**

- **Restricting ovarian mobility**

Laparoscopy is often the only diagnostic tool to uncover this "invisible" cause, and many clients go years without knowing it exists.

Heavy Metal Toxicity and Dental Amalgams

Toxins like **mercury, cadmium, and lead** disrupt:

- **Endocrine signaling**

- **Mitochondrial function**

- **Neural development in embryos**

Mercury from **dental amalgams**, seafood, or industrial exposure has been shown to:

- Cross the placenta

- Impair **sperm morphology** and **egg viability**

- Deplete glutathione (key detox antioxidant)

  Geier et al. (2010) found that stress or teeth grinding significantly increases mercury vapor release from dental amalgams—a silent, cumulative toxic load over time.

Thyroid Dysfunction

The thyroid is **central to fertility**—it regulates metabolic rate, ovulation, and uterine lining thickness. Even **subclinical hypothyroidism** (with "normal" labs) can:

- Disrupt menstrual regularity

- Increase **miscarriage risk**

- Impair **implantation**

Functional range for TSH in fertility is generally **0.5–2.5 mIU/L**, but many patients go undiagnosed when labs use outdated reference ranges.

Hashimoto's Thyroiditis (autoimmune) also interferes with reproductive hormones by triggering **inflammatory responses**, and may be misinterpreted as "unexplained infertility."

Prolactin Imbalance

Hyperprolactinemia inhibits the hypothalamic-pituitary-gonadal axis, suppressing ovulation and libido.

- Causes: **pituitary adenomas, chronic stress, certain antidepressants**

- Symptoms: breast discharge, irregular cycles, low sex drive

Prolactin must be evaluated in patients experiencing **low libido, infertility, or galactorrhea** unrelated to pregnancy or nursing.

Chronic Stress & HPA Axis Dysregulation

Chronic stress is one of the **most underestimated contributors** to infertility:

- Elevates **cortisol**, which **downregulates estrogen, progesterone, and testosterone**

- Impairs **sperm production**

- Causes **anovulation or short luteal phases**

- Dysregulates **blood sugar and insulin**, feeding PCOS-like conditions

The **HPA (hypothalamic-pituitary-adrenal)** axis directly communicates with the reproductive system. If the brain perceives danger, **fertility is shut down as a nonessential function**.

Add to this unresolved emotional trauma—especially reproductive trauma (e.g., miscarriage, abortion, sexual assault)—and the **body may contract against conception**, as a form of subconscious protection.

Beyond Biology: Listening to the Whole Body

Infertility is not always a linear cause-and-effect diagnosis. It is a **multifactorial signal**—an opportunity to slow down, investigate root imbalances, and restore internal harmony. This means asking deeper questions:

- What toxins am I holding—physically and emotionally?

- Where does my body feel safe? Where does it feel restricted?

- Am I nourished, or just fed?

- Is my reproductive system out of balance, or is my entire

ecosystem under strain?

When we widen the lens from conception to connection —to the **connection with self, environment, ancestors, nourishment, and nervous system**—we open new doorways to healing.

Case Study: Marisol & the Mystery of Unexplained Infertility

Marisol, a 35-year-old Afro-Latina professional, had spent three years trying to conceive. After multiple rounds of IUI and IVF, doctors labeled her with "unexplained infertility." Her labs revealed:

- Elevated homocysteine (14.2 umol/L)
- Subclinical hypothyroidism (TSH: 3.1 mIU/L)
- MTHFR C677T mutation

Her holistic protocol included:

- Methylated B-complex vitamins
- Castor oil packs and abdominal massage
- Chelation support with cilantro, chlorella, and NAC (N-acetylcysteine)
- Pelvic floor therapy and trauma-informed somatic counseling

Within eight months, Marisol's homocysteine dropped, her cycles normalized, and she conceived naturally. The shift came not only from physical interventions but from releasing the emotional burden of shame and failure.

Environmental & Lifestyle Factors

In the journey toward fertility, the environment we live in and the lifestyles we lead are not peripheral—they are **central to reproductive health**. Every day, we are exposed to chemicals, habits, and modern-day stressors that disrupt the intricate hormonal dance required for conception. Many of these influences are silent, cumulative, and easily overlooked in conventional reproductive care. Yet when viewed through a holistic lens, they often hold the missing pieces to the fertility puzzle.

Endocrine Disruptors: The Invisible Saboteurs

Endocrine disruptors are chemicals that **interfere with hormone production, binding, and regulation**. They mimic, block, or alter natural hormonal signals, especially estrogen, testosterone, and thyroid hormones—directly impacting reproductive function in both men and women.

Common culprits include:

- **BPA (Bisphenol A):** Found in plastic bottles, canned food linings, and receipts

- **Phthalates:** Present in fragrances, shampoos, lotions, and vinyl materials

- **Parabens:** Used as preservatives in cosmetics and personal care products

- **Pesticides and herbicides:** Common in non-organic produce and household sprays

- **Flame retardants (PBDEs):** Found in furniture, mattresses, and electronics

  Studies have linked exposure to these chemicals with **lower sperm count, ovulatory dysfunction, endometriosis**, and even **increased miscarriage risk** (Diamanti-Kandarakis et al., 2009).

Poor Nutrition: The Fertility-Depleting Diet

The standard Western diet—rich in processed foods, refined sugars, and inflammatory oils—is **antithetical to hormone harmony**. Fertility is a nutrient-intensive process, requiring adequate levels of vitamins, minerals, healthy fats, and amino acids to support egg and sperm development, hormonal cycles, and uterine health.

Key Fertility-Damaging Foods:

- **Sugar and refined carbs:** Promote insulin resistance, a driver of PCOS and anovulation

- **Inflammatory oils (canola, soybean, corn):** Disrupt cell membranes and promote oxidative stress

- **Excess caffeine and alcohol:** Deplete B vitamins, impair liver detoxification, and stress the adrenals

Micronutrients vital for fertility:

- **Folate (not folic acid):** Supports methylation and neural development

- **Zinc:** Crucial for sperm motility and egg quality

- **Vitamin D:** Modulates ovulation, immunity, and progesterone levels

- **Omega-3s:** Support cervical fluid production, reduce inflammation, and balance prostaglandins

  What we eat **literally becomes the building blocks** of the eggs, sperm, and uterine lining. Fertility is fueled by nourishment, not just calories.

Sleep Disruption: Undermining Reproductive Rhythms

Sleep is not just rest—it's **biochemical restoration.** Poor sleep habits disrupt melatonin, cortisol, and insulin levels, all of which are intimately tied to reproductive health.

Melatonin, known for its role in sleep regulation, is also a powerful **antioxidant found in the follicular fluid of ovaries**. It protects developing eggs from oxidative damage and supports the luteal phase of the menstrual cycle (Tamura et al., 2012).

Sleep deprivation may result in:

- Irregular cycles or amenorrhea

- Shortened luteal phase

- Reduced sperm concentration and motility

- Decreased libido and emotional resilience

    One study found that women who slept fewer than 6 hours per night were 25% less likely to conceive than those who got 7–8 hours consistently (Wise et al., 2018).

Fertility-Supportive Sleep Hygiene:

- Go to bed by 10–10:30 PM to align with circadian rhythms

- Reduce blue light exposure in the evening (use amber glasses or screen filters)

- Create a cool, dark, tech-free bedroom sanctuary

- Use herbal allies like chamomile, passionflower, or magnesium glycinate if needed

The Bottom Line

Our environment is not neutral—it is **either supporting or sabotaging fertility every day**. When clients are empowered to reduce toxic exposure, nourish their bodies, and restore circadian alignment, hormonal resilience follows.

Reproductive health is not just about ovulation and semen analysis—it's about living in harmony with the natural design of our biology.

Clinical Application: Translating Insight into Action

Understanding the role of environmental and lifestyle toxins is only half the equation. The real transformation happens when clients are **empowered with clear, actionable strategies** that support detoxification and protect hormone health. As clinicians, educators, and advocates, we can guide clients toward sustainable changes that create safer, more supportive internal and external ecosystems for conception and overall vitality.

1. Encourage Clients to Use Glass or Stainless Steel Containers

Plastic food and beverage containers often leach **Bisphenol A (BPA)** and other estrogen-mimicking chemicals, especially when heated or scratched. These **xenoestrogens** contribute to estrogen dominance, hormone imbalances, and impaired reproductive function.

Why it matters:

- BPA exposure has been linked to **reduced egg quality**, **lower sperm concentration**, and **early miscarriage** (Hunt et al., 2012).

- Reusable glass or stainless steel containers reduce toxic load and are a long-term investment in endocrine safety.

Client Tips:

- Replace plastic water bottles with stainless steel or glass options.

- Never microwave food in plastic containers—opt for

glass or ceramic.

- Store leftovers in glass containers, especially hot or acidic foods.

2. Choose Fragrance-Free, Paraben- and Phthalate-Free Body Products

Many commercial cosmetics, shampoos, lotions, and deodorants contain **endocrine-disrupting chemicals** (EDCs) such as **parabens** (preservatives) and **phthalates** (used to stabilize fragrance).

Why it matters:

- These compounds are absorbed through the skin and **accumulate in fat tissues**, impacting hormone signaling.

- Phthalates have been associated with **low testosterone**, **ovarian dysfunction**, and even **developmental toxicity** in fetuses (Meeker et al., 2009).

Client Tips:

- Read labels: look for "phthalate-free," "paraben-free," and "fragrance-free."

- Encourage use of clean beauty apps like **Think Dirty** or **EWG's Healthy Living** to scan product safety.

- Recommend natural alternatives—such as shea butter, coconut oil, or essential-oil-based deodorants.

3. Switch to Organic, Non-Toxic Cleaning and Pest Control

Household cleaners, air fresheners, and pesticides are often loaded with **volatile organic compounds (VOCs)**, synthetic fragrances, and endocrine-disrupting agents that can accumulate in the liver, lungs, and reproductive tissues.

Why it matters:

- Repeated exposure can contribute to **detoxification overload**, disrupting hormonal clearance pathways.

- Indoor air pollution from cleaners is a major source of **toxic burden** that often goes unrecognized.

Client Tips:

- Swap out bleach-based or ammonia products for natural alternatives like **vinegar, baking soda, and essential oils.**

- Use non-toxic brands like **Branch Basics, Dr. Bronner's, or Seventh Generation.**

- Avoid chemical air fresheners—diffuse essential oils or use natural beeswax candles instead.

4. Advocate for Detoxification Support: Sauna, Liver-Supportive Herbs, and Lymphatic Movement

The body's ability to process and eliminate toxins depends on the **health of the liver, kidneys, skin, lymph, and gut**. Supporting these organs helps regulate estrogen metabolism, eliminate heavy metals, and reduce inflammation.

Why it matters:

- Hormones are detoxified primarily through the **liver's Phase I and Phase II pathways**, especially estrogen.

- Sluggish detox can lead to **hormone recycling**, contributing to conditions like **estrogen dominance**, fibroids, and PMS.

Supportive Interventions:

- **Sauna therapy:** Infrared or traditional sauna use increases sweat-mediated detoxification and boosts circulation.

- **Liver-supportive herbs:**

  o *Milk thistle* (Silybum marianum): Protects liver cells and enhances glutathione production.

  o *Dandelion root*: Stimulates bile flow for estrogen and toxin excretion.

  o *Burdock root*: Aids in purification of the blood and lymph.

- **Nutritional cofactors:** B-complex vitamins, magnesium, selenium, zinc, and N-acetylcysteine (NAC) are critical for Phase II liver detox pathways.

- **Lymphatic movement:** Encourage rebounding (mini-trampoline), dry brushing, or gentle yoga to move stagnation and support drainage.

"Detoxification isn't a one-time event—it's a daily lifestyle of conscious reduction, nourishment, and movement." — Dr. Deilen Michelle Villegas

Visual: Root Causes of Infertility Map

Category	Common Triggers	Impact on Fertility
Hormonal	Thyroid, prolactin, stress, insulin	Irregular cycles, poor egg/sperm quality
Structural	Fibroids, adhesions, pelvic scars	Implantation issues, fallopian blockage
Environmental	Heavy metals, plastics, toxins	Endocrine disruption, oxidative stress

| Genetic | MTHFR mutation, autoimmune conditions | Miscarriage risk, methylation issues |
| Emotional | Trauma, grief, and relationship stress | Nervous system dysregulation |

Disparities in Infertility Diagnosis and Treatment

Infertility does not affect all communities equally. Despite similar or even higher rates of infertility among Black, Indigenous, and People of Color (BIPOC), these individuals are significantly less likely to receive timely diagnosis, access treatment options like Assisted Reproductive Technology (ART), or be heard when voicing reproductive concerns. This disparity is not merely statistical—it is systemic, cultural, and deeply embodied.

Systemic Barriers to Care

Studies consistently show that BIPOC individuals:

- Are **less likely to be referred to fertility specialists**, even after reporting symptoms or trying to conceive for over a year.

- Are **more likely to be misdiagnosed**, especially when they report pain, irregular cycles, or hormonal symptoms—often dismissed as stress-related or minimized entirely.

- Are **underrepresented in clinical trials**, leading to a lack of data on how fertility medications or interventions impact these populations.

- Are **less likely to be offered egg preservation, IVF, or surgical exploration** due to provider bias, socioeconomic assumptions, or institutional racism (Chandra et al., 2013).

Even when BIPOC individuals *do* access fertility care, they face higher out-of-pocket costs, fewer culturally competent providers, and medical systems that often fail to acknowledge the intersection of race, gender, trauma, and reproductive autonomy.

Cultural Stigma and Emotional Silence

In many communities of color, infertility remains a **silent grief**—buried under generational shame, religious expectation, or cultural myths about fertility (e.g., the belief that Black and Latinx women are inherently hyper-fertile). This can leave individuals feeling isolated, ashamed, or "less than" for struggling with something that society has told them should come easily.

Common barriers include:

- Fear of judgment from family or community

- Religious teachings that discourage assisted reproduction

- Internalized pressure to be "strong" or not show vulnerability

- Lack of representation in fertility narratives, media, or advocacy

A Holistic, Culturally-Aware Approach

As clinicians and healers, it is critical to:

- **Validate reproductive grief** as a real and multidimensional trauma—not just about physical loss, but emotional identity, ancestral pressure, and life path disruption.

- **Acknowledge the historical wounds** that shape distrust in the medical system (e.g., forced sterilizations, the Tuskegee Study, medical experimentation on enslaved Black women).

- **Integrate cultural and spiritual frameworks** into healing—honoring traditions, ancestors, and rituals around fertility, womb care, and the sacredness of conception.

- **Offer trauma-informed fertility counseling** that makes room for both tears and hope, both science and spirit.

Reproductive Justice is Holistic Justice

We cannot speak of fertility without also speaking of access, agency, and autonomy. Reproductive justice, as coined by Black women leaders in the 1990s, calls for **the right to have children, not have children, and raise children in safe and healthy environments.** This includes the right to receive quality fertility care, to grieve reproductive loss without stigma, and to make empowered decisions about one's body—regardless of race, gender identity, or income level.

> "Fertility is not just physical—it is also emotional, ancestral, and energetic." – Dr. Villegas

Fertility & Compatibility: The Hidden Dynamics of Conception

In the realm of human reproduction, the journey to conception is more than the sum of eggs, sperm, and ovulation timing. While traditional fertility assessments often focus on individual biomarkers—such as hormone levels, ovarian reserve, or sperm motility—**a growing body of research points to a deeper truth**: fertility is also shaped by the **biochemical dialogue between two bodies.** It's not just about whether the reproductive systems work, but whether they work *together.*

Just as chemistry influences attraction, **biological compatibility plays a role in conception, implantation, and pregnancy maintenance.** Certain couples, despite being healthy as individuals, may face unexplained infertility due to underlying immunological or genetic mismatch—an often overlooked but critical component of fertility medicine.

The Role of Genetic Compatibility

At the center of this hidden dance is the **Major Histocompatibility Complex (MHC)**—a group of genes responsible for immune system regulation. In humans, this system is known as the **Human Leukocyte Antigen (HLA) complex.**

- Research suggests that **greater genetic diversity in HLA types between partners is linked to higher fertility rates and better pregnancy outcomes** (Roberts et al., 2008).

- Couples with **too-similar HLA profiles** may experience difficulty conceiving, increased miscarriage risk, or implantation failure. This is because the immune system may fail to properly recognize the embryo as a "semi-foreign" entity, leading to a lack of appropriate tolerance or immune support during early pregnancy.

In essence, our **innate biology seeks novelty and diversity at the genetic level**, favoring pairings that enhance offspring immunity and long-term vitality. This echoes ancient evolutionary wisdom: diversity isn't just beautiful—it's biologically intelligent.

Sperm-Egg Communication: More Than Meets the Eye

Fertilization isn't a passive process. Eggs release **chemoattractants**, which act as biological signals that help guide compatible sperm toward them. Recent studies show that:

- **Eggs may selectively attract sperm from genetically preferred partners**, even in vitro.

- This phenomenon, sometimes called **"cryptic female choice,"** reveals that fertility is not simply mechanical —it is relational at the cellular level (Løvlie & Pizzari, 2019).

This suggests that the **egg "communicates" with sperm** in search of the best genetic match, and that subtle incompatibilities—unseen by traditional testing—may disrupt this communication.

Immunological Tolerance and Maternal Acceptance

Pregnancy requires the **maternal immune system to accept the embryo,** which carries foreign paternal antigens. This delicate balance of immune activation and suppression must be precisely modulated.

Some couples experience **recurrent pregnancy loss (RPL)** or **implantation failure** due to:

- **Antiphospholipid antibodies**

- **Natural Killer (NK) cell overactivation**

- **Unregulated cytokine activity**

- **Lack of proper maternal-fetal tolerance**

In such cases, **immunological testing** may reveal the need for interventions like:

- Lymphocyte Immunization Therapy (LIT)

- Low-dose steroids or intralipids

- Dietary and herbal immunomodulation

- Mind-body practices to reduce systemic inflammation

The Energetic and Emotional Dimension of Compatibility

From a holistic perspective, fertility also reflects the **energetic synergy between two people**. Ancient medicine systems like Chinese Medicine, Ayurveda, and Shamanic traditions teach that conception requires **alignment of heart, mind, and energy** between partners.

- Is there mutual safety, love, and openness?

- Are emotional wounds or power imbalances creating subtle blocks?

- Is the conception being forced or flowing?

Energetic mismatches—emotional tension, lack of intimacy, unresolved trauma—can create **invisible resistance** in the conception process, even when all labs appear normal. **The womb listens. The body remembers.**

Clinical Takeaway: Compatibility Matters

For couples facing unexplained infertility, recurrent miscarriage, or IVF failure, consider exploring:

- HLA compatibility testing

- Sperm DNA fragmentation analysis

- Immunological screening (cytokines, NK cells, antiphospholipid antibodies)

- Energetic counseling and relationship alignment

- Somatic therapies to release emotional and relational trauma

  "Sometimes, the block to conception isn't within the individual—but within the connection." — Dr. Deilen Michelle Villegas

Genetic Compatibility and Cryptic Female Choice

The human reproductive system is far more intelligent and selective than we often give it credit for. While conventional science once framed fertilization as a race of sperm to the egg, new research reveals a far more sophisticated and **collaborative** interaction between gametes—especially driven by the **female reproductive system**.

At the center of this theory lies the concept of **Cryptic Female Choice (CFC)**—a biological process through which a female's body exerts subtle, often unconscious control over which sperm succeeds in fertilizing her egg. Originally observed in non-human species, CFC suggests that **the female reproductive environment can "favor" sperm from genetically compatible partners**, even post-ejaculation.

The Science Behind CFC in Humans

Emerging research supports the notion that **ovarian follicular fluid and cervical mucus can influence sperm motility, survival, and selection.** In a 2020 study by Fitzpatrick et al., it was found that sperm from certain men swam better in the follicular fluid of specific women—**not necessarily their partners—indicating a hidden biological preference based on genetic compatibility.**

Key mechanisms potentially involved in this gamete-level selection include:

- **Immune signaling molecules** in cervical and uterine fluids that respond more favorably to compatible sperm

- **Molecular receptors on the egg's zona pellucida (outer shell)** that exhibit selective binding affinity

- **Variations in HLA (Human Leukocyte Antigen) profiles**, which may influence the immune acceptance of sperm and embryo

This means fertilization is not purely a numbers game—it's also a **genetic negotiation** between two sets of biological codes, with the female body playing gatekeeper for optimal genetic fitness.

Why Compatibility Matters: Beyond Just Conception

Cryptic female choice isn't simply about fertilization—it's about **ensuring the healthiest potential for offspring**. By selecting sperm that offers the greatest immunological and genetic diversity (especially in HLA genes), the female reproductive system helps:

- Enhance **embryo viability**

- Reduce **risk of miscarriage**

- Strengthen **offspring immune function**

- Optimize **maternal tolerance of pregnancy**

In couples where conception is challenging despite normal fertility markers, **incompatibility at this invisible level may be at play**. While this does not make a couple "incompatible" in the emotional or spiritual sense, it does suggest that **conception may require greater biological synergy, immunomodulation, or assisted guidance** to align both partners' systems.

Implications for Fertility Counseling and Treatment

Understanding CFC can revolutionize how we approach unexplained infertility, IVF failures, or recurring miscarriages. It also reframes the narrative: **not all fertility challenges originate from pathology—some reflect natural biological selectivity.**

Clinical Considerations:

- **HLA compatibility testing** may be useful for couples with recurrent pregnancy loss

- IVF with intracytoplasmic sperm injection (ICSI) may bypass natural gamete-level selection—but could increase the risk of immune-related rejection

- Functional medicine can support **immune modulation and mucosal health** to optimize the uterine environment for natural selection processes

- Emotional and somatic work can resolve **subconscious relational, sexual, or energetic resistance**, allowing the body to open more fully to conception

A Holistic Reflection: The Womb Knows

From a metaphysical perspective, cryptic female choice aligns with ancient teachings about the **womb as a sentient organ** —one that discerns not only who we create with, but **how aligned that creation is with our soul, safety, and purpose.**

In energetic healing traditions:

- The womb is seen as the seat of **intuition, generational memory, and creative power**

- Unconscious resistance to a partner, unresolved trauma, or ancestral wounding may all influence **fertility and receptivity**

- CFC is not just a physical process—it is a **biological expression of feminine wisdom**

  "The body doesn't just want to create life—it wants to create aligned, thriving life." — Dr. Deilen Michelle Villegas

Immunological Compatibility and HLA Matching

Pregnancy is a biologically extraordinary phenomenon—it requires the mother's immune system to **tolerate and support** an embryo that is, by genetic standards, half foreign. Central to this immune negotiation is the **Human Leukocyte Antigen (HLA) system**, a group of proteins encoded by genes that help the immune system recognize self from non-self.

HLA molecules, found on nearly every cell in the body, serve as cellular ID tags. They play a crucial role in determining immune tolerance, transplantation success, and—more subtly —influencing fertility and pregnancy outcomes.

The Role of HLA in Fertility and Implantation

In reproductive immunology, HLA compatibility between partners has emerged as a **significant factor in conception and miscarriage rates**. While moderate compatibility ensures immune harmony, **excessive HLA similarity can signal danger to the maternal immune system**, particularly during the critical stages of embryo implantation and placental development.

When HLA Similarity Becomes a Problem:

- The embryo may fail to trigger adequate **immune-modulating responses** from the maternal system.

- This can result in **weak trophoblast invasion**, impaired placental formation, or **failure to establish immune tolerance**, leading to implantation failure or miscarriage.

- Essentially, the mother's body may not "recognize" the embryo as a semi-foreign entity needing protection and support.

Conversely, **HLA dissimilarity—especially within the HLA-C and HLA-G genes—has been associated with:**

- Stronger **maternal-fetal immune dialogue**

- Healthier **placental development**

- Increased **live birth rates**, particularly in couples with a history of unexplained infertility or recurrent pregnancy loss

  "Conception isn't just a physical union—it is an immunological negotiation. And sometimes, that negotiation breaks down in silence." — Dr. Deilen Michelle Villegas

Clinical Implications of HLA Matching

HLA testing is not routinely offered in standard fertility clinics, yet it holds immense potential for:

- Couples experiencing **recurrent miscarriages**

- Cases of **unexplained infertility** despite normal labs

- Failed **implantation in IVF or IUI cycles**

Testing involves genotyping both partners to determine the

degree of HLA similarity, particularly focusing on:

- **HLA-C (class I molecules)**: Associated with NK (natural killer) cell activation and implantation response

- **HLA-G (class Ib molecules)**: Critical for establishing maternal tolerance of the fetus

- **KIR (killer immunoglobulin-like receptors)**: Found on maternal NK cells and determine how they respond to fetal HLA-C

Couples with high HLA compatibility or "unfavorable" KIR/HLA combinations may benefit from **immune-modulating therapies**, such as:

- Low-dose **aspirin or prednisone** to reduce inflammation

- **Intravenous immunoglobulin (IVIG)** or **intralipids** to balance immune responses

- Functional medicine support for gut immunity and inflammatory regulation

Holistic Lens: The Body as Oracle

From an integrative perspective, the **womb is not just a physical space—it's a deeply intelligent environment.** When conception doesn't occur despite structural and hormonal health, **the immune system may be signaling a lack of alignment, safety, or readiness** on a deeper level.

Energetic, emotional, or ancestral considerations include:

- Unresolved grief or trauma stored in the **sacral chakra** or **pelvic floor**

- Energetic cords to past partners that influence reproductive receptivity

- Subconscious fears or inherited beliefs around motherhood, birth, or relationship trust

- Inherited immune system "memories" that may still be activated from previous generational experiences (e.g., miscarriage, loss, infertility trauma)

Integrative Support Options

To support couples with HLA-related fertility challenges, practitioners can incorporate a **whole-body, whole-being approach:**

Clinical + Holistic Strategies:

- Immune balancing with **omega-3s, turmeric, NAC, and glutathione**

- Gut microbiome healing (a strong gut-immune connection improves reproductive outcomes)

- Reiki or womb healing to process stored trauma

- EMDR or somatic therapy for fear of loss or failed conception

- Couples' work to process emotional pain and strengthen relational safety

- Spirit baby connection practices to create space for new life energetically

  "Sometimes, conception is not about trying harder —but about aligning more deeply." — Dr. Deilen Michelle Villegas

Antisperm Antibodies and Partner-Specific Immune

Responses

In the intricate dance of human reproduction, the immune system plays a far more active—and sometimes disruptive—role than we often acknowledge. One of the lesser-known contributors to infertility is the development of **antisperm antibodies (ASA),** which can interfere with a couple's ability to conceive, even when all other reproductive markers appear normal.

What Are Antisperm Antibodies?

Antisperm antibodies are **immune proteins (IgA, IgG, or IgM)** produced by the body in response to the presence of sperm. While sperm is naturally immunogenic (recognized as foreign due to its unique protein markers), it is typically protected from immune detection by the **blood-testis barrier** and immunosuppressive factors within the female reproductive tract.

However, when this immune tolerance is disrupted—through infection, trauma, sexual injury, inflammation, or unknown causes—the immune system may begin to **recognize sperm as a threat** and mount an attack.

These antibodies can:

- **Bind to sperm** and impair motility (preventing forward movement)

- **Agglutinate sperm** (cause them to stick together)

- **Block sperm receptors**, reducing the ability to penetrate cervical mucus or fertilize the egg

- Trigger local inflammation or immune rejection at the site of fertilization

Partner-Specific Immune Reactions: When

Compatibility Becomes Immunological

What makes this phenomenon even more complex is that **ASA reactions can be highly partner-specific**. In some cases, a woman may produce antisperm antibodies **only in response to one specific partner's sperm**, while remaining immunologically tolerant to sperm from another partner. This points to a deeper, individualized immunological interaction— where the combination of two people's immune systems may either support or hinder conception.

Such reactions may involve:

- **HLA incompatibilities** (as explored in the previous section)

- Unique **seminal fluid proteins** triggering immune reactivity

- Preexisting **mucosal inflammation** or dysbiosis in the vaginal or endocervical canal

- **Sexual trauma**, which can create subconscious or physiological barriers to receptivity

This immunological mismatch can lead to unexplained infertility, especially when structural, hormonal, and timing factors appear optimal.

Testing for ASA and Immune Compatibility

Testing for antisperm antibodies can be done via:

- **Postcoital test (PCT)**: Assessing sperm motility in cervical mucus after intercourse

- **MAR (Mixed Antiglobulin Reaction) test** or **Immunobead test**: Identifying sperm-bound antibodies in semen or cervical fluids

- **Serum testing**: Measuring circulating ASA in blood

Additionally, advanced fertility clinics may offer **partner-specific immunological testing**, particularly in cases of recurrent pregnancy loss or repeated IVF failure.

Clinical and Holistic Strategies for Immune-Related Infertility

When ASA or partner-specific immune responses are suspected, integrative protocols can help reduce inflammation, promote immune tolerance, and optimize reproductive health.

Conventional Interventions:

- **Corticosteroids** to suppress immune reactivity (short-term use)

- **Intrauterine insemination (IUI)** to bypass cervical mucus

- **IVF with sperm washing** to reduce exposure to antigens

Integrative & Holistic Support:

- **L-glutamine, zinc, and omega-3s** to repair mucosal barriers

- **Probiotics** to restore vaginal and cervical microbiome health

- **Liver and lymphatic detoxification** to aid immune regulation

- **Womb massage, castor oil packs, or Mayan abdominal therapy** to reduce pelvic inflammation

- **Energy healing, EFT tapping, or somatic therapy** to address trauma-based immune responses to intimacy or conception

> "Sometimes, it's not that the body is broken—but that it is protecting itself from an unprocessed story. Fertility requires safety, not just function." — Dr. Deilen Michelle Villegas

Implications for Fertility Treatments and Counseling

In the realm of fertility care, unexplained infertility often leaves couples navigating a fog of frustration, confusion, and grief. Yet in many of these cases, the issue may not lie within the individual, but in the **unique biochemical and immunological interaction between partners**. Understanding partner compatibility—particularly at the genetic and immune system levels—offers a powerful key to decoding this mystery and reimagining how we approach fertility treatment and counseling.

Personalized Assessment Beyond Standard Protocols

Traditional fertility evaluations tend to focus on:

- Hormonal panels

- Semen analysis

- Ovulation tracking

- Uterine and tubal imaging

While these are essential, they often **exclude immune and compatibility-based assessments** unless there is a history of recurrent miscarriage or failed IVF attempts.

Integrating evaluations for:

- **HLA compatibility**

- **Antisperm antibodies**

- **Cytokine and inflammatory profiles**

- **Natural killer (NK) cell activity**

- **Microbiome imbalances in reproductive tissue**

can shift the treatment trajectory from trial-and-error to **precision-guided fertility care.**

Genetic Compatibility and Counseling

When genetic mismatches such as high HLA similarity or MTHFR gene mutations are identified, couples can be counseled on how these factors:

- Influence embryo implantation

- Affect maternal immune tolerance

- May require more tailored interventions, such as **immunomodulatory therapies**, **embryo screening**, or **donor-assisted reproduction**

This knowledge also empowers couples to make informed, compassionate decisions about their reproductive journey— **removing the burden of self-blame** and reframing infertility as a complex interaction, not a personal failure.

Emotional & Relational Dimensions of Compatibility Counseling

The psychological toll of repeated unsuccessful fertility treatments is immense. By introducing compatibility-based frameworks into counseling, practitioners can help couples:

- Rebuild a sense of hope and direction

- Understand that "unexplained infertility" may have underlying biological validity

- Explore **alternative routes to parenthood** (e.g., donor sperm/egg, surrogacy) with clarity rather than shame

- Strengthen emotional intimacy by acknowledging the shared nature of the challenge

"When compatibility is addressed with compassion, couples move from blame to bonding. It's not about who's at fault—it's about what the body needs to feel safe enough to conceive." — Dr. Deilen Michelle Villegas

Clinical Pathways Forward

Depending on the compatibility profile, providers might consider:

- **Immunotherapy protocols** (e.g., intralipid infusions, IVIG)

- **Endometrial receptivity analysis** to tailor embryo transfer timing

- **Partner-specific timed insemination** to reduce immune reactivity

- **Preconception detox and immune reset programs**

- **Somatic co-regulation work** for couples to repair relational safety on a physiological level

Bridging Science and Soul in Fertility Counseling

The concept of partner incompatibility can be devastating at first—but it can also offer profound clarity. It shifts the narrative from "broken body" to **"complex partnership,"** where healing becomes a shared, empowered journey. Fertility practitioners must be equipped to hold both the **clinical science** and the **emotional landscape** of these revelations.

Couples need:

- **Spiritual and energetic support** to process grief or pivot toward new paths

- **Culturally sensitive care** that honors ancestral, emotional, and relational influences on fertility

- **Long-term wellness planning**, including hormone recovery and trauma-informed sexual reconnection

Embracing the Complexity of Human Reproduction

Human reproduction is not a linear equation. It is an **intricate dance of biology, emotion, chemistry, energy, and timing**. The path to conception cannot be reduced to ovulation charts, semen counts, or textbook hormone ranges. It is a multidimensional process shaped by a constellation of factors —**some visible, others hidden beneath the surface of medical checklists and cultural expectations**.

While conventional fertility models focus heavily on individual pathology, emerging science invites us to **shift the lens**: not just asking "what is wrong with the individual," but "what is happening between the individuals?" Compatibility —**genetic, biochemical, and immunological**—matters. A couple's unique interaction may determine not only whether conception occurs, but whether a pregnancy is sustained, whether the body feels safe, and whether reproductive energies align.

This recognition doesn't complicate the fertility journey—it **liberates it**.

It opens the door to:

- **More precise diagnostics** that validate lived experiences of infertility even when standard labs are "normal"

- **Holistic treatment pathways** that honor the body's need for alignment, not just intervention

- **Compassionate counseling** that supports both partners in releasing shame and stepping into empowered decision-making

As practitioners and individuals alike, embracing this complexity means **moving beyond blame** and into curiosity. It means holding space for science and soul, data and intuition, medicine and mystery. It's about understanding that **fertility is not a guarantee—it is an ecosystem**, and every ecosystem must be nourished in its own way.

> "Every body tells a story, and every couple writes a new chapter. When we stop seeing infertility as failure, and start seeing it as a call to deeper attunement, healing begins." — Dr. Deilen Michelle Villegas

Let us reframe infertility—not as a final verdict, but as **an invitation**:

- To listen more closely to the body's whispers

- To explore not just the "how," but the "why"

- To reconnect with one another, not just as reproductive beings, but as emotional, energetic, and spiritual partners on the journey of life creation

A Return to Wholeness

Infertility is never just about the reproductive organs—it is a message. A signal. A sacred whisper from the body inviting us to **slow down, listen, and re-align**. While modern medicine often isolates the problem to hormone panels, ovulation timing, or sperm count, true healing asks us to widen the lens. **Infertility is not a failure of function—it is an invitation to deeper integration.**

We must remember: the body is not broken; it is **responding** —to stress, to trauma, to inflammation, to toxicity, to disconnection. When we stop viewing conception as a linear process and begin to see it as a *confluence of physical readiness, emotional safety, relational harmony, and spiritual alignment,* we open the door to **wholeness.**

Healing infertility is not just about:

- Stimulating ovaries or increasing sperm motility

- Reducing inflammatory markers

- Taking the "right" supplements
  It's also about:

- Releasing stored grief and generational trauma from the womb

- Restoring trust in the body after medical or emotional violation

- Rekindling intimacy beyond performance or pressure

- Realigning one's life with cycles of rest, nourishment, pleasure, and vitality

"When we return to wholeness, we don't just make space for a baby—we make space for new life in all its forms." — Dr. Deilen Michelle Villegas

This return to wholeness may include:

- **Somatic healing** to release blockages from pelvic trauma or stored shame

- **Functional medicine testing** to decode silent imbalances

- **Partner communication rituals** to rebuild safety and co-regulation

- **Womb-centered spiritual practices** to reconnect with feminine power

- **Honoring the grief and uncertainty** of the path without losing hope

When we cultivate an internal and external ecosystem of **safety, vitality, and trust**, the body often responds—not always with immediate pregnancy, but with a deeper sense of healing, embodiment, and peace. From that foundation, conception—biological or otherwise—can occur with **integrity rather than desperation.**

This is not the bypassing of pain, but the **transformation of it**.

This is not about fixing the body.
This is about **listening to it**.

References

Berker, B., Kaya, C., Aytac, R., Satiroglu, H., & Mollamahmutoglu, L. (2009). Homocysteine concentrations in follicular fluid are associated with poor oocyte and embryo qualities in polycystic ovary syndrome patients undergoing IVF. *Journal of Assisted Reproduction and Genetics, 26*(10), 591–596. https://doi.org/10.1007/s10815-009-9354-0

Geier, D. A., Kern, J. K., & Geier, M. R. (2010). The relationship between mercury and autism: A comprehensive review and discussion. *Journal of Toxicology and Environmental Health, Part B, 13*(7–8), 511–529. https://doi.org/10.1080/10937404.2010.483736

Bjordahl, T. S., Lu, C., & Milne, G. (2021). Cryptic female choice: A review of the literature and implications for human fertility. *Philosophical Transactions of the Royal Society B: Biological Sciences, 376*(1835), 20200174. https://doi.org/10.1098/rstb.2020.0174

Hedrick, P. W., & Black, F. L. (1997). HLA and mate selection: No evidence in South Amerindians. *American Journal of Human Genetics, 61*(3), 505–511. https://doi.org/10.1086/515510

Ober, C. (1999). Studies of HLA, fertility and mate choice in a human isolate. *Human Reproduction Update, 5*(2), 103–107. https://doi.org/10.1093/humupd/5.2.103

Pinto, S., Luddi, A., Governini, L., Morgante, G., Piomboni, P., & De Leo, V. (2018). Antisperm antibodies and fertility: Clinical significance and therapeutic approaches. *Journal of Assisted Reproduction and Genetics, 35*(10), 1839–1850. https://doi.org/10.1007/s10815-018-1261-4

van der Horst, F. A., & Maree, D. J. F. (2014). Immunological causes of infertility. *Obstetrics and Gynaecology Forum, 24*(4), 35–39. https://hdl.handle.net/10520/EJC160620

CHAPTER 7

Modern Day Infertility —
Lifestyle Therapy as Medicine

Reclaiming Fertility through Root-Cause Healing

In today's fast-paced, toxic, and overstimulated world, infertility is no longer just a clinical concern—it has become a **cultural epidemic**. But the deeper truth is this: **infertility is not the body's betrayal—it is its wisdom.** The body does not shut down its reproductive capacity without reason. It conserves, protects, and adapts in response to its environment, and when it perceives that environment as unsafe, unstable, or depleted, it puts reproduction on pause.

> "What is labeled 'infertility' is often the body saying, 'I don't feel safe enough to create life." -- Dr. Deilen Michelle Villegas

Through a **root-cause approach**, we shift from simply "trying to get pregnant" to asking *why the body has chosen not to conceive.* When we approach fertility through this lens, the goal is no longer to manipulate or override the body—but to **listen to it, nourish it, and support it back to optimal function**.

Common Modern Disruptors to Fertility:

- **Chronic Stress & Burnout**
  Prolonged cortisol elevation impairs ovulation, lowers libido, depletes progesterone, and disrupts the hypothalamic-pituitary-gonadal (HPG) axis. The body interprets survival mode as incompatible with reproduction.

- **Inflammatory & Processed Diets**
  Diets high in refined sugar, trans fats, gluten, and dairy can inflame the gut lining, elevate insulin levels, and throw off sex hormone balance. Blood sugar instability alone can cause anovulation and impair egg quality.

- **Gut Dysbiosis & Microbiome Imbalance**
  A compromised gut affects nutrient absorption, estrogen detoxification, and immune signaling. The estrobolome (gut bacteria involved in estrogen metabolism) is key to hormonal harmony.

- **Environmental Toxins & Endocrine Disruptors**
  Xenoestrogens found in plastics, synthetic fragrances, pesticides, and personal care products mimic or block natural hormones, leading to estrogen dominance, thyroid disruption, and low sperm count.

- **Unprocessed Trauma & Nervous System Dysregulation**
  Somatic memory stored in the pelvic floor and womb space can block energetic and physiological flow. Birth trauma, reproductive grief, or sexual violation can suppress reproductive function subconsciously.

Lifestyle Therapy as a Sacred Prescription

Lifestyle therapy isn't just behavior change—it is **ritualized reclamation.** It's how we re-teach the body that it is safe to rest, to receive, and to create. Here's how:

1. Nervous System Regulation

Daily breathwork, vagus nerve toning, and somatic practices help downshift from sympathetic survival mode to parasympathetic restoration. This is the foundation of hormonal healing.

2. Nourishment Over Dieting

Focus on anti-inflammatory, fertility-supportive foods:

- Healthy fats (avocado, flax, wild-caught salmon) for hormone production

- Cruciferous vegetables (broccoli, kale) for estrogen detox

- B vitamins, zinc, selenium, and magnesium for egg and sperm health

3. Toxic Load Reduction

- Use glass or stainless-steel containers

- Switch to clean beauty and household products

- Filter water and avoid plastic-wrapped or microwaved food

4. Gut & Liver Support

- Incorporate probiotics and fermented foods

- Use herbs like dandelion, burdock root, and milk thistle to assist detox

- Support regular elimination (bowel movements, sweating, lymphatic drainage)

5. Restorative Movement

Trade excessive cardio or HIIT for fertility-friendly options like:

- Walking in nature

- Yin yoga

- Rebounding or Pilates

These help increase circulation to the pelvis and reduce cortisol levels.

6. Energetic Womb Healing

- Womb massage or abdominal therapy

- Guided visualizations and emotional release

- Yoni steaming or castor oil packs for uterine nourishment and detox

Healing, Then Conceiving

The body was designed to conceive. When it doesn't, it's not failing—it's **waiting. Waiting for alignment. Waiting for nourishment. Waiting for you to come home to it.**

When we stop "fighting" infertility and start *honoring* it as a signal of deeper imbalance, healing becomes possible—and from healing, life can emerge.

> "Fertility is not a linear formula. It is the flowering of a well-tended ecosystem." — Dr. Deilen Michelle Villegas

Environmental Estrogens and Endocrine Disruption

In our modern world, one of the most overlooked yet powerful contributors to hormonal imbalance—and by extension, infertility—is the constant exposure to **environmental estrogens**, also known as **xenoestrogens**. These are synthetic or natural chemical compounds that **mimic or interfere with the body's endogenous estrogen** by binding to estrogen receptors and disrupting the delicate endocrine balance that governs reproductive, metabolic, and neurological health.

Unlike natural estrogen, which follows the body's cyclical rhythm, xenoestrogens **linger in tissues**, accumulate over time, and signal the body in unpredictable and often harmful ways. This **disrupts the estrogen-progesterone relationship**, leads to **estrogen dominance**, and has been linked to a **surge in reproductive disorders, early puberty, reduced fertility, and hormone-driven cancers.**

Common Xenoestrogen Sources in Daily Life:

Source	Examples
Plastics & Packaging	BPA, BPS, phthalates in plastic containers, water bottles, food wrap
Canned Foods	Epoxy resin linings in cans leach BPA into food
Personal Care Products	Parabens, sulfates, triclosan in shampoos, lotions, deodorants, toothpaste
Makeup & Skincare	Synthetic fragrances and preservatives in cosmetics
Household Cleaners	Surfactants, synthetic scents, and industrial solvents
Non-Organic Produce	Pesticide residues—particularly atrazine, DDT derivatives, glyphosate
Receipts and Thermal Paper	High BPA content absorbed through skin
Furniture and Mattresses	Flame retardants (PBDEs) linked to hormone disruption

	and fetal harm
Tap Water	Residues of birth control pills, industrial waste, and pharmaceuticals

What the Research Shows:

1. **Reproductive Health Impacts:**

   o Xenoestrogen exposure has been linked to:

      - **Anovulation**

      - **Reduced sperm motility and count**

      - **Ovarian dysfunction and PCOS**

      - **Uterine fibroids and endometriosis flare-ups**

   o (Diamanti-Kandarakis et al., 2009; Meeker & Ferguson, 2011)

2. **Hormonal Development & Puberty:**

   o Increased exposure during early childhood or in utero is associated with:

      - **Precocious puberty in girls**

      - **Altered gender expression and reproductive development in boys**

      - **Increased lifetime risk of hormone-related cancers**

3. **Fetal and Epigenetic Effects:**

   o   In utero exposure can alter **gene expression via epigenetic imprinting**, affecting multiple generations.

   o   Disruption of maternal-fetal hormone communication can lead to lifelong metabolic and neurological challenges.

How Xenoestrogens Disrupt the Endocrine System:

- **Estrogen Receptor Binding**: They bind to estrogen receptors in the absence of actual estrogen, leading to overstimulation.

- **Inhibition of Hormone Metabolism**: They can impair detoxification enzymes in the liver, leading to recirculation of estrogen.

- **Disruption of Feedback Loops**: By mimicking estrogen, they trick the hypothalamus and pituitary into downregulating natural hormone production.

- **Thyroid Suppression**: Many xenoestrogens also interfere with thyroid hormone receptors, affecting metabolism and fertility.

- **Impact on the Gut-Liver Axis**: They affect the **estrobolome**, the gut bacteria involved in estrogen detoxification.

Clinical Implications & Counseling Tips:

Clients struggling with infertility, PCOS, endometriosis, fibroids, or menstrual irregularities should be **screened for**

environmental exposures as part of a root-cause evaluation.

Key questions to assess:

- What kinds of containers do you store or reheat food in?

- What personal care products do you use daily?

- Is your water filtered? Do you drink from plastic bottles?

- Do you regularly consume non-organic produce or processed food?

- Are you exposed to synthetic scents (candles, air fresheners, perfumes)?

Detox and Recovery Approaches:

1. Environmental Detox:

- Eliminate plastic containers—use **glass, stainless steel, or ceramic.**

- Choose **fragrance-free, paraben- and phthalate-free** personal care and cleaning products.

- Prioritize **organic produce** and animal products to reduce pesticide and hormone exposure.

- Install **water and air filters** to reduce chemical load.

2. Liver & Hormonal Detoxification Support:

- **Cruciferous vegetables** (broccoli, kale, Brussels sprouts) boost liver enzyme pathways.

- **Supplements**: DIM (diindolylmethane), calcium-D-glucarate, NAC, and milk thistle.

- **Dry brushing, infrared saunas, castor oil packs**, and **lymphatic massage** to mobilize stored toxins.

3. Gut Health & Elimination:

- Ensure **daily bowel movements**—fiber, magnesium, and probiotics are foundational.

- Support gut lining with **L-glutamine, collagen, and omega-3s.**

4. Hormonal Rebalancing:

- Monitor **estradiol, estrone, estriol**, and estrogen metabolites via DUTCH or saliva testing.

- Rebuild progesterone via stress reduction, B6, magnesium, and herbal allies like **Vitex**.

   "Environmental estrogens are invisible saboteurs of reproductive vitality. But awareness is the first step toward sovereignty." — Dr. Deilen Michelle Villegas

We must not only cleanse our bodies—but also reimagine our environments as sanctuaries of hormonal balance, nourishment, and life-giving energy.

Gut Dysbiosis: The Microbiome-Fertility Connection

We often speak of the gut as the "second brain," but in fertility work, it may also be considered the **"second womb."** The state of the gut microbiome profoundly influences reproductive health, not just through digestion, but by **regulating hormones, managing inflammation, supporting detoxification, and training the immune system.** When the gut is out of balance—also known as **dysbiosis**—the entire hormonal landscape can become destabilized, creating an internal environment inhospitable to conception and implantation.

"Fertility isn't just about the ovaries—it's a reflection of the gut, the liver, the immune system, and the entire ecosystem of the body." — Dr. Deilen Michelle Villegas

How the Microbiome Impacts Fertility:

1. **Hormone Metabolism and Detoxification:**

   o The **estrobolome**, a specialized community of gut bacteria, produces **β-glucuronidase**, an enzyme that determines whether estrogen is excreted or reabsorbed.

   o If dysbiosis leads to **overactive β-glucuronidase**, estrogen that should be eliminated is reabsorbed, fueling **estrogen dominance, fibroids, endometriosis**, and **PMS**.

   o Liver detox pathways are also impaired without sufficient **microbial diversity**, leading to **hormonal congestion**.

2. **Nutrient Absorption:**

   o Key fertility nutrients such as **iron, zinc, magnesium, selenium, B12, folate, and vitamin D** depend on gut health for absorption.

   o Dysbiosis or inflammation compromises the **intestinal lining**, reducing uptake and creating hidden deficiencies that sabotage egg and sperm quality.

3. **Immune System Regulation:**

○ Up to **70% of the immune system resides in the gut.**

○ When dysbiosis occurs, the **gut lining becomes permeable (leaky gut)**, releasing endotoxins (LPS) that trigger **autoimmune activation**, which can result in **embryo rejection, implantation failure**, or **miscarriage.**

4. **Inflammatory Load:**

○ An imbalanced microbiome increases **pro-inflammatory cytokines** (e.g., IL-6, TNF-α), contributing to **chronic low-grade inflammation.**

○ This chronic inflammation disturbs ovulation, impairs progesterone production, and affects sperm morphology and motility.

Common Signs of Dysbiosis in Fertility Clients:

- Bloating, gas, or irregular stools (IBS, constipation, diarrhea)

- Recurrent yeast infections, BV, or urinary tract infections

- Skin conditions: eczema, acne, rosacea

- Food intolerances or multiple sensitivities

- Brain fog, anxiety, or chronic fatigue

- History of antibiotic use, birth control pills, or PPI (acid blocker) medication

These are not isolated symptoms—they are **invitations to look deeper** into the gut as a root cause of fertility struggles.

The Estrobolome: Guardian of Hormonal Balance

The **estrobolome** is a dynamic group of gut microbes that specifically regulates **estrogen metabolism**. When this subset is disrupted:

- **Estrogen recirculates**, intensifying estrogen-dominant conditions (e.g., PCOS, fibroids, endometriosis)

- Detox pathways become sluggish, leading to **PMS, mood swings, breast tenderness**, and **cycle irregularity**

- Reproductive immune signaling becomes distorted, increasing the likelihood of **implantation failure**

Clinical Integration: Supporting Gut Health for Fertility

Step 1: Functional Testing

- **Comprehensive stool analysis (GI-MAP, GI Effects)**

- **Zonulin, calprotectin, and LPS antibodies** to assess gut permeability

- **β-glucuronidase levels** to evaluate estrogen recycling

- **Candida/yeast overgrowth** and pathogenic bacterial markers

Step 2: Targeted Protocols

- **Phase 1: Remove** harmful bacteria, yeast, or parasites using botanicals (e.g., oregano oil, berberine, caprylic acid)

- **Phase 2: Replace** enzymes, hydrochloric acid (if needed), and bile salts

- **Phase 3: Rebuild** the gut lining with L-glutamine, aloe vera, zinc carnosine

- **Phase 4: Re-inoculate** with high-quality probiotics and prebiotic fibers

- **Phase 5: Rebalance** lifestyle factors: stress, sleep, and nutrition

Step 3: Dietary Foundations

- Increase fiber-rich foods: **flaxseed, chia, leafy greens, root vegetables**

- Emphasize **fermented foods** (if tolerated): sauerkraut, kefir, kimchi, miso

- Eliminate known triggers: **gluten, dairy, sugar, alcohol**, and **processed seed oils**

- Support bile flow and liver function with **beets, dandelion, artichoke**, and **milk thistle**

Somatic & Nervous System Considerations

Gut dysfunction is often exacerbated by **sympathetic dominance**—when the body is stuck in "fight or flight." Incorporate:

- **Vagus nerve stimulation** (humming, gargling, cold exposure)

- **Somatic grounding practices**

- **Breathwork and meditation** to reduce inflammation and

enhance parasympathetic tone

> "The gut doesn't just digest food—it translates environment, emotion, and energy into biochemistry. To heal the womb, we must first heal the terrain." — Dr. Deilen Michelle Villegas

Rebalancing the microbiome is not a trend—it's a **clinical imperative** in restoring fertility, vitality, and whole-body coherence.

PCOS, Endometriosis & the Inflammatory Loop

Polycystic Ovary Syndrome (PCOS) and endometriosis are often treated as isolated reproductive disorders. However, a deeper, systems-based perspective reveals that both are **manifestations of chronic internal imbalance**, particularly involving **inflammation, metabolic dysfunction, and immune dysregulation.** Their presence signals a complex interplay between the endocrine, immune, and digestive systems—highlighting the need for root-cause healing over symptom suppression.

> "These conditions aren't the body's betrayal—they're its cry for rebalance." — Dr. Deilen Michelle Villegas

Understanding PCOS: A Metabolic-Endocrine Imbalance

PCOS is not a single disease—it is a **syndrome** with various expressions and phenotypes. While many associate it with polycystic ovaries seen on ultrasound, the true dysfunction lies in:

- **Hyperandrogenism:** Elevated testosterone and DHEA levels that can cause acne, hirsutism, and anovulation.

- **Insulin Resistance:** The majority of individuals with

PCOS exhibit impaired glucose tolerance and elevated insulin, which in turn stimulates androgen production from the ovaries.

- **Anovulation and Menstrual Irregularity:** Chronic lack of ovulation leads to irregular or absent periods, impacting fertility.

Root Triggers:

- **Refined sugar and processed carbohydrates** creating insulin spikes

- **Chronic stress and cortisol elevation**, contributing to adrenal androgen excess

- **Xenoestrogens and obesogens** from plastics, cosmetics, and food packaging disrupting hormone signaling

Understanding Endometriosis: A Wound of the Immune & Hormonal Systems

Endometriosis is a **highly inflammatory and estrogen-driven condition** in which endometrial-like tissue grows outside the uterus—on the ovaries, fallopian tubes, intestines, or pelvic lining. This causes:

- **Chronic pelvic pain**

- **Inflammation and adhesions**

- **Ovulatory dysfunction and poor egg quality**

- **Heightened risk of miscarriage and implantation failure**

Root Triggers:

- **Estrogen dominance**, often worsened by poor detoxification pathways and xenoestrogen exposure

- **Gut permeability and immune activation**, allowing inflammatory mediators to trigger widespread pelvic inflammation

- **Epigenetic trauma and somatic holding**, particularly when tied to sexual trauma, grief, or unresolved ancestral pain

The Inflammatory Feedback Loop

Both PCOS and endometriosis participate in a **self-reinforcing inflammatory loop:**

1. **Insulin resistance or poor detoxification** leads to hormonal imbalance.

2. Hormonal imbalance (especially excess estrogen or androgens) **triggers tissue changes** and immune activation.

3. The immune system, in an attempt to regulate damage, **produces more cytokines and prostaglandins**, increasing pain, bloating, and fatigue.

4. Ongoing inflammation worsens metabolic and hormonal dysfunction—creating a cycle that continues unless interrupted by systemic intervention.

Integrative Healing: Rebalancing the Terrain

True healing for PCOS and endometriosis requires a **multi-layered lifestyle medicine approach**, which supports the endocrine, immune, detoxification, digestive, and nervous systems.

1. Anti-Inflammatory Nutrition

- Emphasize:

  - Wild-caught fish, flaxseeds, walnuts (**omega-3s**)

  - Cruciferous vegetables (broccoli, cauliflower, Brussels sprouts) for **estrogen detox**

  - Turmeric, ginger, rosemary, garlic for anti-inflammatory support

  - High-fiber foods to support hormone elimination

- Reduce/Eliminate:

  - Dairy, gluten (particularly in endometriosis)

  - Sugar, refined carbs

  - Processed seed oils and inflammatory snacks

2. Insulin Sensitivity & Blood Sugar Regulation

- Key supplements:

  - **Myo-inositol & D-chiro inositol** (restore ovulation and reduce insulin resistance)

  - **Berberine** (natural insulin sensitizer and antimicrobial)

  - **Magnesium, chromium,** and **alpha-lipoic acid** for

glucose balance

- Lifestyle:

  o Time-restricted eating or gentle intermittent fasting

  o Movement after meals to stabilize glucose (e.g., walking, yoga)

3. Liver & Lymphatic Detoxification

- Support Phase I/II liver detox with:

  o **Milk thistle, N-acetylcysteine (NAC), DIM, calcium-D-glucarate**

- Dry brushing, rebounding, castor oil packs to promote lymphatic drainage

- Deep breathing and movement to assist estrogen clearance

4. Somatic & Emotional Regulation

- Address the **nervous system component** of these conditions:

  o Somatic therapy to release pelvic tension and stored trauma

  o Breathwork and vagus nerve activation to reduce inflammation

  o Emotional release around themes of unworthiness, grief, or reproductive identity

Case Reflection: Leah's Recovery Journey

Leah, a 29-year-old with a PCOS diagnosis, came in after years of birth control use and difficulty conceiving. She struggled with cystic acne, sugar cravings, and irregular cycles. Her lab work showed high insulin, elevated DHEA, and low progesterone.

Together, we:

- Removed refined sugar and dairy

- Introduced **berberine**, **magnesium glycinate**, and **inositol**

- Implemented **castor oil packs** and **gentle cycle-syncing movement**

- Explored body image trauma and childhood stress through somatic journaling and EMDR

Within 6 months, her cycles returned, and she conceived naturally on her 7th cycle—after 3 years of "infertility."

"Healing the womb begins with listening to the wisdom of inflammation—not silencing it. When we decode the signal, the body will lead us home." — Dr. Deilen Michelle Villegas

Detoxification as a Fertility Pathway

Detoxification isn't about punishment, deprivation, or crash cleanses. It's about *clearing the clutter*—both physical and energetic—that interferes with the body's natural intelligence. In the realm of fertility, detoxification becomes a sacred act of preparation: **making space for life to enter**. Before conception can occur, the internal terrain must be safe, balanced, and welcoming.

"We don't just conceive in the womb—we conceive through the bloodstream, the tissues, and the mind. Detoxification makes conception possible by restoring harmony in the places we don't often see."
— Dr. Deilen Michelle Villegas

Why Detoxification Matters for Fertility

In today's toxic environment, our bodies are constantly burdened by a **daily load of chemicals, hormone disruptors, and inflammatory triggers** that were never meant to be part of our internal landscape. These toxins accumulate in our fat cells, circulate through our blood, and disrupt hormone metabolism, ovulation, egg and sperm quality, and implantation.

Toxins can:

- Mimic or block sex hormones (xenoestrogens, heavy metals)

- Inhibit liver enzymes required for hormone clearance

- Disrupt gut bacteria that regulate estrogen elimination (estrobolome)

- Increase systemic inflammation and immune dysregulation

- Cause oxidative stress that damages DNA in sperm and eggs

True detoxification supports the **organs of elimination**—*liver, kidneys, lymphatic system, colon, lungs, and skin*—and enhances the body's ability to restore equilibrium.

Clinical Detox Strategies for Preconception Health

A well-structured detox is **gentle, targeted, and supportive**, aiming to nourish and empower the body rather than deplete it.

Phase I/II Liver Support

The liver metabolizes hormones and neutralizes toxins via two key phases of detoxification:

- **Phase I**: Breaks down toxins using enzymes dependent on **B vitamins** and antioxidants

- **Phase II**: Conjugates (binds) those metabolites for elimination, supported by **glutathione, amino acids, sulfur-rich foods**, and **milk thistle**

Key Nutrients & Herbs:

- **B-complex vitamins** (especially B6, B12, folate)

- **Glutathione** or NAC (precursor)

- **Milk thistle, dandelion root, turmeric, artichoke extract**

Binders for Toxin Capture

Binders help trap toxins in the gut and escort them out before they are reabsorbed into circulation (a common problem in those with sluggish digestion).

Examples:

- **Activated charcoal** (binds chemicals and endotoxins)

- **Chlorella** (chelates heavy metals and supports mitochondria)

- **Bentonite clay** (binds mold toxins and estrogens)

Lymphatic Movement & Drainage

The lymphatic system, unlike the circulatory system, **has no pump**. It relies on movement and manual techniques to move waste from tissues to detox organs. Stagnant lymph = inflammation and toxic overload.

Recommended Practices:

- **Rebounding (mini trampoline)** for 10–15 minutes daily

- **Dry brushing** before showers to stimulate lymph flow

- **Castor oil packs** over the liver or womb area to reduce inflammation and support drainage

- **Manual lymphatic massage** when available

Sweat, Hydration & Bowel Regularity

Sweating is one of the **most effective ways** to excrete heavy metals, phthalates, and BPA.

Key Recommendations:

- **Infrared sauna sessions** 2–3 times per week (if tolerated)

- **Daily hydration** with filtered water + pinch of sea salt or trace minerals

- **Regular elimination** (1–3 bowel movements/day) to prevent hormone recirculation

- **Magnesium citrate, flaxseed**, or **triphalā** for natural constipation relief

Gentle Detox Protocols: Nourish to Eliminate

A holistic fertility detox is never about starvation—it's about

nourishment for elimination.

Detox plans should include:

- **Warm, fiber-rich foods**: Stews, soups, cruciferous vegetables, legumes

- **Daily greens**: Arugula, dandelion, parsley, cilantro (bile movers + blood purifiers)

- **Healthy fats**: Avocado, olive oil, coconut oil (support cell membranes + hormone production)

- **Protein**: Clean, organic sources to support Phase II liver pathways

Additional Integrative Supports

- **Coffee enemas** (for liver stimulation and glutathione boost)

- **Epsom salt baths** (magnesium replenishment and muscle relaxation)

- **Breathwork + vagus nerve activation** (to downshift the nervous system and support digestive flow)

- **Adaptogenic herbs** (ashwagandha, schisandra, holy basil) to reduce cortisol and support resilience

Case Study: Nadia's Renewal

Nadia, a 32-year-old South Asian woman, presented with PCOS, acne, fatigue, and absent ovulation for over a year. She had been placed on birth control in her teens and underwent multiple rounds of Clomid with no success. Her intake revealed chronic constipation, a high-stress lifestyle, and regular use of commercial beauty products.

Her holistic plan included:

- Switching to non-toxic personal care and household products
- Daily fiber and probiotic intake
- Blood sugar regulation via nutrient-dense meals and gentle intermittent fasting
- Nervous system support through breathwork and restorative movement

By month six, Nadia's cycle returned, ovulation was confirmed via BBT charting, and she reported improved skin and energy. Her fertility returned as her body felt safe, nourished, and balanced.

Case Study: Talia's Fertility Reset

Talia, a 34-year-old client with unexplained infertility, presented with irregular cycles, PMS, fatigue, and a history of mold exposure and processed food dependence. Hormone testing revealed estrogen dominance, high cortisol, and sluggish liver enzymes.

Her **8-week fertility detox** included:

- Binders (chlorella + bentonite clay)

- Daily rebounding + castor oil packs

- Liver support (milk thistle, NAC, turmeric)

- Anti-inflammatory diet with cruciferous veggies, flax, and bone broth

- Emotional release through womb journaling and somatic healing

By week six, her bloating had reduced, her sleep improved, and her cycle regulated. Four months later, she conceived naturally —with the first truly pain-free period she'd had in years.

Visual: Modern Infertility Root Contributors

Root Cause	Symptoms/Impact	Lifestyle Solution
Xenoestrogens	Hormone disruption, estrogen dominance	Detox products, switch to clean living
Gut Dysbiosis	Bloating, poor hormone clearance	Probiotics, fiber, fermented foods
PCOS/Endometriosis	Irregular cycles, pain, inflammation	Anti-inflammatory diet, insulin support
Stress	Ovulation suppression, cortisol dysregulation	Nervous system work, adaptogens

Lifestyle as the Foundation for Conception

Infertility is not a sentence—it's a signal. It is not a personal defect or a biological betrayal, but rather the body's profound intelligence communicating that the internal environment is not yet safe for creation. The body does not deny life out of failure; it pauses it out of protection.

> "The body never works against us—it speaks in symptoms, delays, and imbalances to redirect us toward healing." — Dr. Deilen Michelle Villegas

In a culture that often seeks quick fixes and interventions, we must return to the deeper truth: **fertility is not separate from overall health**. It is the outcome of balance—hormonal, emotional, nutritional, spiritual. And balance begins with lifestyle.

The Internal Terrain: Is it Safe to Conceive Here?

The human body is exquisitely designed to prioritize survival. When it detects chronic stress, inflammation, poor nutrient reserves, or toxic burden, it wisely downregulates fertility as a protective mechanism. From a biological standpoint, the womb will not open to life if it senses that the environment is too hostile to sustain it.

Conditions that tell the body it's unsafe to conceive:

- Blood sugar dysregulation and insulin resistance

- Inflammatory markers like CRP and IL-6

- Excess cortisol and flattened diurnal rhythms

- Nutrient depletion (iron, B12, zinc, iodine, magnesium)

- Gut dysbiosis and malabsorption

- Xenoestrogen exposure disrupting hormonal feedback loops

When we address these imbalances **at the root**, the body often responds by restoring ovulation, regulating cycles, enhancing libido, and improving egg and sperm quality—without the need for invasive interventions.

The Power of Lifestyle Medicine

1. Restore the Gut

- The gut is where nutrient absorption, immune tolerance, estrogen metabolism, and inflammation regulation begin.

- Healing the gut can reduce autoimmunity, support progesterone production, and improve egg and sperm vitality.

- Support includes: fermented foods, diverse fibers,

prebiotics/probiotics, and GI repair nutrients like glutamine and zinc carnosine.

2. Detox the Environment

- Endocrine disruptors (BPA, phthalates, parabens) mimic hormones and confuse the body's delicate feedback systems.

- Lifestyle shifts like using non-toxic body products, glass containers, and clean air/water drastically reduce this burden.

3. Regulate the Nervous System

- Chronic stress signals the HPA axis to suppress reproduction.

- Cortisol competes with progesterone production and shortens the luteal phase.

- Somatic healing, breathwork, rest, joy, and emotional safety are *fertility medicine.*

4. Honor Circadian Rhythms

- Hormones are released on a light-dark cycle. Poor sleep and artificial light exposure blunt melatonin and disrupt the hypothalamic-pituitary-ovarian (HPO) axis.

- Fertility-enhancing practices include: early morning sunlight, screen curfews, magnesium baths, and sleep hygiene rituals.

5. Move with Intention

- Gentle, consistent movement (walking, yoga, strength training) improves insulin sensitivity, circulation to reproductive organs, and lymphatic drainage.

- Avoid overtraining, which can suppress ovulation and elevate cortisol.

A Return to Biological Wisdom

Fertility does not bloom in chaos. It emerges in environments where the body feels nourished, resourced, and safe.

We must ask:

- *Is there enough nourishment here—physically, emotionally, spiritually—for new life to flourish?*

- *Am I planting seeds in soil that has been truly tended to, or in terrain that's been neglected and depleted?*

Fertility is not just about cycles and ovulation—it's about *wholeness*. When we begin to live in alignment with nature's rhythms, our own biology follows suit. The womb reawakens. Hormones recalibrate. Vitality returns.

Reframing the Journey

This is not just a lifestyle "intervention"—it's a lifestyle *invitation*. An opportunity to come home to your body. To nourish it with consistency, compassion, and care. To see your fertility not as a monthly countdown, but as a **vital sign** of your overall wellness.

> "Conception is not just about becoming a parent —it's about becoming a vessel for creation. And that begins with how we live, breathe, and nourish ourselves every day." — Dr. Deilen Michelle Villegas

References

Diamanti-Kandarakis, E., Bourguignon, J. P., Giudice, L. C., Hauser, R., Prins, G. S., Soto, A. M., ... & Gore, A. C.

(2009). Endocrine-disrupting chemicals: An Endocrine Society scientific statement. *Endocrine Reviews, 30*(4), 293–342. https://doi.org/10.1210/er.2009-0002

Institute for Functional Medicine. (2022). *Functional medicine approach to reproductive health.* Retrieved from https://www.ifm.org

CHAPTER 8

Menopause & Mortality —
The Unspoken Transition

The Second Initiation

Menopause is not a medical failure. It is not a curse to be cured or a pathology to be pacified. It is the *second initiation*— a sacred unraveling of what no longer serves, so that a deeper, more sovereign version of the self can emerge.

In the dominant cultural narrative, menopause is synonymous with loss: loss of youth, loss of desirability, loss of hormones, vitality, identity. This deficit-based lens reduces the menopausal body to a shell of its former function, framing the end of menstruation as the death of usefulness. But within ancestral wisdom traditions, **menopause is not an ending—it is an elevation.**

> "Menopause is not the end of womanhood—it is the birth of a new archetype." — Dr. Deilen Michelle Villegas

Where the maiden initiated the journey, and the mother sustained it, the **crone** or **wise woman** completes the sacred triad. She becomes the embodied portal of inner knowing, fierce boundaries, spiritual maturity, and collective memory. This transition is not only hormonal—it is spiritual, neurological, emotional, and deeply existential.

The Modern Disconnect

Western medicine often defines menopause by its symptoms —hot flashes, night sweats, mood changes, vaginal dryness —rather than its meaning. It medicalizes the transition, prescribing hormones without addressing the deeper transformation that is unfolding underneath.

Yet what if the discomforts were not just dysfunctions, but *messages*? What if the heat of a hot flash was not just a biological reaction, but the fire of internal alchemy—burning away what no longer belongs?

Our ancestors didn't fear menopause. They revered it. In many cultures, women who had crossed the threshold of fertility were considered spiritually potent and politically powerful. Their wisdom was sought, their intuition honored, their presence vital.

Today, too many women enter this phase unprepared, unsupported, and unseen—taught only to manage the symptoms, not to honor the transformation.

Menopause as Alchemy: The Inner Fire

Biochemically, menopause is characterized by the decline of estrogen and progesterone, changes in cortisol regulation, shifts in brain plasticity, and an increased demand on the adrenal glands. These physiological changes are real—and they are substantial.

But what if these hormonal changes are not just signs of decline... but the opening of a new energetic frequency?

Estrogen withdrawal awakens deeper self-reflection.
Progesterone decline stirs the emotional waters and sharpens intuition.
Cortisol sensitivity forces us to confront our stress thresholds and restructure our lives.
Oxytocin drops challenge us to cultivate internal connection, rather than outsourcing worth.

Menopause is not passive. It is *initiatory*. It demands confrontation—with our mortality, with our regrets, with our truth. And if we answer the call, it rewards us with wisdom, sovereignty, and clarity unlike any other life stage.

The Archetype of the Wise Woman

In this second initiation, we move from being the nurturer of others to becoming the guardian of our inner flame. We reorient our lives around integrity, not obligation. Around peace, not people-pleasing. Around alignment, not appeasement.

This is the time of:

- **She who says no without apology**

- **She who remembers what was silenced**

- **She who mentors, protects, and preserves**

- **She who bleeds no more, but births wisdom**

The womb may no longer release blood, but it now holds *legacy*.

Honoring the Transition

This phase deserves ritual. Ceremony. Integration. Reflection. Just as we celebrate first bleeds and births, we must also *honor the last bleed* as a moment of spiritual completion and rebirth.

Practices to honor the second initiation:

- Create a **"Womb Farewell"** ceremony—write a letter to your body, release shame, and express gratitude for all it has carried.

- Engage in **crone circles**—intergenerational spaces for storytelling, embodiment, and wisdom transmission.

- Support the nervous system with **somatic rituals**, **adrenal nourishment**, **herbal allies** (like black cohosh, maca, ashwagandha), and **restorative movement**.

- Reclaim pleasure and sensuality not through youth, but through presence, self-intimacy, and energetic radiance.

- Explore creative pursuits that have long been suppressed. This is the era of *voice*, *vision*, and *volition*.

> "The second initiation teaches us to lead not from fertility, but from frequency—not from production, but from presence." — Dr. Deilen Michelle Villegas

Menopause is not the death of womanhood. It is the death of pretending, performing, and proving. It is the resurrection of the true self. Of the woman who no longer bleeds, yet births truth with every word she speaks.

Understanding Perimenopause: The Overlooked Passage

Perimenopause is the *silent upheaval* of womanhood—the bridge between cycles and stillness, vitality and reinvention. And yet, in the world of clinical care, it remains wildly misunderstood, underdiagnosed, and emotionally invalidated.

While menopause is often marked by the final menstrual period, **perimenopause** is the *years-long hormonal unraveling* that precedes it—and it can feel like being pulled into the undercurrent without a map, language, or lifeline.

> "Perimenopause is not just the road to menopause— it is the awakening before the rebirth." — Dr. Deilen Michelle Villegas

The Hormonal Chaos Beneath the Surface

Perimenopause typically begins in the mid-to-late 30s

(sometimes earlier), extending into the mid-40s and beyond. Ovarian function becomes erratic. Estrogen may spike unpredictably, then plummet. Progesterone—already delicate —often declines more dramatically. Testosterone may trickle downward or remain constant, creating confusing shifts in desire, energy, and emotional bandwidth.

What results is a hormonal seesaw, where **internal chaos exists without external validation**. You're not "old enough" for menopause, yet no longer hormonally stable. You may still be fertile, but your cycles are unreliable. You feel exhausted, weepy, irritable, electric, numb—sometimes in a single day.

Common Symptoms of Perimenopause (That Are Often Misdiagnosed):

- **Irregular or heavy menstrual cycles:** Estrogen dominance without enough progesterone to balance it

- **Hot flashes, night sweats, chills:** Vasomotor instability as thermoregulation falters

- **Sleep disruption and chronic fatigue:** Declining melatonin and cortisol rhythm dysregulation

- **Mood swings, memory fog, and anxiety:** Estrogen fluctuations impact serotonin, dopamine, and GABA levels

- **Vaginal dryness and libido loss:** Lower estrogen and testosterone affect lubrication, sensation, and desire

- **Acne, dry skin, and thinning hair:** Hormonal imbalances impact sebum production and collagen synthesis

The Identity Crisis No One Talks About

Perimenopause often coincides with one of the busiest seasons of life: raising children, building careers, navigating relationships, caregiving for aging parents. The internal shifts are profound—but invisible. You may look "fine" on the outside, yet inside, you are unraveling, awakening, reassembling.

Sexual desire may feel unpredictable or nonexistent—not from disinterest, but from disconnection. The physical body may feel foreign. Emotions become harder to regulate. And without context, **many women internalize their symptoms as personal failure rather than physiological transition.**

This invisibility leads to misdiagnosis (e.g., antidepressants for hormonal mood swings), gaslighting (from partners or providers), and isolation (because no one warned us this would happen *this soon*).

Support Strategies for the Perimenopausal Woman

The key to navigating perimenopause isn't suppression—it's *sacred support* and physiological alignment. Here's how we begin:

Hormone Testing

- DUTCH testing or salivary panels can identify estrogen dominance, progesterone deficiency, cortisol rhythms, and androgens

- Avoid guessing; test to understand the *specific dance* of your hormones

Adaptogenic and Nervous System Support

- **Maca**, **ashwagandha**, **shatavari**, and **rhodiola** can help buffer adrenal burnout and stabilize mood

- **Magnesium glycinate** and **vitamin B6** support

progesterone and reduce irritability

Cycle Syncing

- Adjust lifestyle, exercise, and nutrition to the phase of your shifting cycle

- This creates internal coherence and reduces hormonal resistance

Somatic and Mind-Body Therapies

- Perimenopause triggers old emotional patterns stored in the body

- Incorporate **breathwork, vagal toning, EMDR,** or **trauma-informed movement**

Therapeutic Conversations & Cultural Healing

- Work with practitioners who validate this transition as a whole-body, whole-self process

- Join women's circles, therapy groups, or intergenerational dialogues to reclaim this narrative

Reframing Perimenopause as Initiation

What if this isn't a breakdown—but a **breaking open?**

What if your irritability is a boundary rising?
Your fatigue a divine nudge to rest?
Your memory lapses an invitation to release what no longer needs remembering?

Perimenopause is not a flaw in your femininity. It is *the refining fire*—the holy shedding of old hormones, old identities, and outdated expectations. It asks you to slow down, listen inward, nourish deeply, and **rewrite the definition of womanhood** on your own terms.

"This is not the end of your vitality—it is the beginning of your authority." — Dr. Deilen Michelle Villegas

Men, Fertility, and the Illusion of Youth

A striking and persistent pattern appears across cultures and generations: as men age, many begin to gravitate toward significantly younger partners. This trend—often explained away by biology or preference—is not simply about aesthetics, libido, or fertility. It reveals something much deeper: a collective discomfort with feminine evolution, aging, and embodied power.

In clinical work and cultural analysis alike, this pattern exposes a profound **psychospiritual avoidance** of the depth, discernment, and awakening that often emerges in women during their 40s and beyond.

"When a woman awakens, she becomes impossible to manipulate—and that scares people who only know how to love from control." — Dr. Deilen Michelle Villegas

Youth as Projection, Not Preference

Younger women are often idealized as symbols of vitality, fertility, and flexibility. They are statistically:

- Less likely to be experiencing hormonal shifts like perimenopause

- More likely to be socially conditioned to seek external validation

- Often still forming their personal identity, and less likely to challenge relational power dynamics

In other words, the attraction to younger women is not

purely about beauty—**it is about the illusion of emotional ease**. Youth is perceived as more "manageable," less likely to confront, question, or require profound emotional presence.

But this dynamic reveals a painful truth: **some men are not seeking partnership—they are seeking reflection.** Reflection of their virility, their desirability, their status. A younger woman becomes a mirror that affirms youth, instead of a partner who asks for inner maturity.

The Mature Feminine: Why She Is Often Feared

As women enter perimenopause and move toward menopause, a powerful metamorphosis begins.

They become:

- More embodied, intuitive, and unapologetically vocal

- Less likely to prioritize pleasing others over pleasing themselves

- Spiritually attuned and emotionally precise

- Intolerant of emotional immaturity, dishonesty, or misalignment

This shift threatens relational dynamics built on control, performance, or ego validation. A woman in her second initiation no longer fears her truth—and **she no longer tolerates partners who do.**

To a man who has never confronted his own wounds, shadows, and insecurities, **a woman in her power is not alluring—she is terrifying.**

Men Chasing Youth to Avoid Their Own Aging

In seeking younger partners, many men are not simply trying to "feel young again"—they are *running from the mirror of their own mortality.* To confront a partner in her 40s or 50s who is rising in power, depth, and truth requires a man to rise alongside her.

It requires:

- Emotional regulation and nervous system maturity

- Shadow work and relational accountability

- The capacity to meet depth with depth—not deflection

Without this internal work, many men will continue to seek novelty over intimacy, youth over wisdom, and fantasy over truth.

Rewriting the Relationship Paradigm

This isn't a condemnation of age-gap relationships—some are rooted in mutual respect, emotional maturity, and spiritual alignment. But we must call out the societal tendency to **vilify aging women** while **rewarding aging men** for clinging to youth as a status symbol.

The menopausal and post-menopausal woman is not a discarded version of her younger self—**she is an alchemist**, capable of transmuting pain into wisdom, passion into purpose, and desire into discernment.

> "She no longer seduces from insecurity. She magnetizes from embodiment." — Dr. Deilen Michelle Villegas

Feminine Power Must Be Seen, Not Silenced

When society teaches men to fear emotional intensity, spiritual depth, and mature embodiment, it creates generations of relational dysfunction. Healing this requires cultural and interpersonal shifts:

- **Educate men** on the neurobiology and power of perimenopause and menopause

- **Create relational rites of passage** for aging couples to evolve together

- **Celebrate the wise woman archetype** in media, education, and relationship discourse

- **Encourage therapy, mentorship, and emotional intelligence work for men in midlife**

Men do not have to lose themselves to love a powerful woman. But they *do* have to find themselves.

And when they do—when men awaken to their own depth— they no longer chase youth. They seek resonance. They seek real.

Biological Landscape of Menopause: The Inner Terrain of Transformation

Menopause is not a singular event but a **physiological and spiritual metamorphosis** that spans a decade or more. While mainstream medicine often reduces it to a "loss of hormones," menopause is, in truth, a sacred biological evolution—a shift in hormonal architecture that impacts every system in the body and every facet of the self.

Typically occurring between **ages 45 and 55**, menopause is clinically defined as the absence of menstruation for **12 consecutive months**. But its true beginning often lies years prior, in the tumultuous terrain of **perimenopause**—a hormonal transition phase that may start as early as the **mid-to-late 30s** and last 4–10 years.

Common Physiological Shifts in the Menopausal Transition

1. **Decline in Estrogen & Progesterone (Ovarian Hormones):**

    o   Estrogen regulates cognition, skin elasticity, vaginal health, bone strength, and emotional regulation. As it declines, symptoms like **hot flashes, mood swings, vaginal dryness**, and **joint pain** emerge.

    o   Progesterone, a natural anti-anxiety hormone and sleep aid, declines earlier and faster than estrogen, contributing to **irritability, insomnia**, and a sense of internal restlessness.

2. **Elevated FSH & LH:**

    o   As estrogen declines, the pituitary gland increases **follicle-stimulating hormone (FSH)** and **luteinizing hormone (LH)** in an attempt to stimulate the ovaries. These elevations are often used as diagnostic markers of menopause.

3. **Testosterone & DHEA Drop:**

    o   While produced in smaller amounts than in males, **testosterone** supports libido, muscle tone, drive, and confidence in all bodies. A decline in testosterone and its precursor **DHEA** can result in:

        ▪   Fatigue and brain fog

        ▪   Low sexual desire

        ▪   Reduced resilience to stress

- Decreased sense of motivation or ambition

4. **Neurotransmitter Changes:**

   o Declining estrogen impacts **serotonin, dopamine, and acetylcholine**, which can lead to:

      - Increased anxiety and depressive symptoms

      - Difficulty concentrating

      - Short-term memory lapses

      - Emotional sensitivity

5. **Bone, Heart, and Metabolic Shifts:**

   o Estrogen protects **bone density, cardiovascular health**, and **metabolic function**. Its loss raises the risk of:

      - Osteopenia and osteoporosis

      - Heart disease and high cholesterol

      - Insulin resistance and abdominal weight gain

Beyond Symptoms: The Energetic Reconfiguration

While the biological symptoms of menopause are very real, they are only one layer of the transformation. Underneath the night sweats and mood swings lies a **profound energetic shedding**—a dismantling of who we were in order to reclaim who we are becoming.

> "This is not a breakdown—it is a realignment. The fire in your veins is not dysfunction—it is initiation." — Dr. Deilen Michelle Villegas

Menopause is an alchemical process. The body becomes less hormonally driven by reproduction, and more attuned to preservation, intuition, and wisdom. What emerges is a **rewiring of the nervous system** to support spiritual growth, legacy building, and inner sovereignty.

Reframing the Landscape: From Decline to Design

Too often, menopausal shifts are pathologized as the "loss of womanhood." But what if they are the **architecture of ascension?**

What if the hot flash is the body's way of releasing emotional residue?

What if the mood swing is not mood *dysregulation*, but a call to release buried truths?

What if the fog is not forgetfulness—but a temporary veil as you reorient your perception?

Clinical Tools and Empowered Support

This phase deserves more than hormone prescriptions and dismissive advice. True healing and balance require a **multidimensional approach:**

- **Functional Lab Testing:** DUTCH hormone panels, thyroid function, DHEA, insulin, and cortisol rhythm mapping

- **Herbal Support:** Black cohosh, vitex, maca, dong quai, ashwagandha

- **Nutritional Therapy:** Phytoestrogens, magnesium, B-complex, vitamin D3, omega-3s

- **Mind-Body Tools:** Somatic therapy, yoga nidra, breathwork, guided visualization

- **Spiritual Integration:** Journaling, women's circles, ancestral practices, ritual to honor the shift

An Invitation to Reclaim the Wise Woman Archetype

Menopause is a **second initiation**—from Maiden to Mother, and now from Mother to Mystic. It asks us not to mourn what was, but to **celebrate what is awakening**.

In indigenous and ancestral cultures, this phase was revered. The bleeding ceased not because life was ending, but because the energy once used for physical creation was now available for **spiritual, communal, and creative leadership**.

> "You are not drying up—you are distilling down to your essence." — Dr. Deilen Michelle Villegas

The Mortality Link: Facing the Void

Menopause is more than the end of ovulation—it is an initiation into a new season of life that few are prepared for and even fewer are supported in. When the cycles stop, something deeper begins: an **existential unraveling** that brings mortality to the forefront of consciousness.

In modern society, where youth is worshipped and aging is feared, the menopausal woman often finds herself **unseen**, **misunderstood**, or **discarded**. She is no longer the mother, the maiden, or the object of desire. She is becoming the crone, the mystic, the mirror—and that frightens a culture obsessed with surface.

Hormones, Identity, and the Mirror of Mortality

Biochemically, the brain during menopause undergoes a neuroendocrine shift remarkably similar to puberty—but with one major difference: **puberty is celebrated**, while menopause is pathologized.

- **Estrogen and progesterone** influence not only reproduction but mood, cognition, and emotional regulation.

- Their decline can trigger not only hot flashes and insomnia, but also **existential grief**, identity dissolution, and spiritual disorientation.

- For many, the hormonal shifts stir deep internal questions:

  - *"Who am I if I am no longer fertile?"*

  - *"What do I have to offer if society no longer sees me as desirable?"*

  - *"Am I still a woman if I no longer bleed?"*

These are not signs of psychological breakdown. These are the **spiritual symptoms of awakening**.

> **"This confrontation with 'the void' is not a sign of pathology—it is the medicine."**
> — Dr. Villegas

The "void" is not emptiness. It is the **sacred womb of rebirth**. When approached consciously, this phase becomes a portal to self-knowledge, embodied wisdom, and unapologetic wholeness. The parts of the self that were performative, pleasing, or externally defined begin to die—making room for authenticity and alignment.

Case Study: Anika's Awakening

Anika, a 52-year-old Caribbean-American mother of three, came to therapy overwhelmed by symptoms she couldn't articulate: sudden **panic attacks**, nightly **hot flashes**, **sexual numbness**, and a disconnection from her previously vibrant self. Though her OB/GYN prescribed **HRT**, her symptoms persisted, accompanied by feelings of shame, resentment, and a profound sense of loss.

Through integrative care, we explored the **emotional landscape beneath the hormones**:

- Her youngest had just left for college.

- She felt invisible in her marriage and disconnected from her body.

- She realized her identity had been built on caregiving, and now she was adrift.

Together, we wove a sacred reclamation:

- **Narrative therapy & journaling** allowed her to mourn her past roles and reimagine her next chapter.

- **Black cohosh**, **maca**, and **vitex** supported her endocrine system naturally.

- **Strength training** helped her feel rooted and powerful again, while **yoga nidra** restored rest and nervous system regulation.

- **Somatic sex therapy** helped her access new forms of pleasure and sensuality not tied to performance or reproduction.

After four months, Anika wasn't just sleeping better—she

was *living* differently. She began teaching workshops on empowered aging for women in her community and launched a creative arts project she had shelved for decades. Menopause was no longer a death—it became her resurrection.

Midlife as Metamorphosis, Not Decline

When women enter the portal of menopause, they are metabolizing much more than hormonal shifts:

- **Grief over aging parents**

- **Loneliness in long-term relationships**

- **Disappointment in unmet dreams**

- **Awakening to inner callings once silenced by responsibility**

Rather than suppress these feelings with pharmaceuticals alone, we must treat menopause as a **psycho-spiritual passage** —one that calls for **ritual, reverence, and redefinition**.

Reframing the Void as Vision

In indigenous traditions, the menopausal woman becomes the **spiritual matriarch**, the dreamkeeper, the community's source of truth. Her intuition sharpens. Her energy, once cycled outward through menstruation, now turns inward, becoming a force of vision and clarity.

Let us teach women that:

- **Their power does not end—it concentrates.**

- **Their body is not betraying them—it is rebalancing.**

- **Their voice is not too loud—it is finally being heard.**

"You are not disappearing. You are distilling into your most essential form." — Dr. Deilen Michelle Villegas

Hormone Therapy and Functional Alternatives

Modern medicine often frames menopause as a hormonal deficiency, positioning hormone replacement therapy (HRT) as the primary or only solution. While **bioidentical or pharmaceutical HRT** can offer profound relief for some—particularly those navigating severe hot flashes, insomnia, and vaginal atrophy—it is not without risks and is not universally suitable. The truth is, **there is no one-size-fits-all roadmap for menopause**, because no two women carry the same story, physiology, or healing journey.

Instead, many women are turning to **functional and integrative strategies** to support the transition with gentleness, agency, and wisdom—reclaiming their hormonal sovereignty through nourishment, lifestyle, and sacred self-tending.

"Menopause is not a malfunction to be fixed—it is a recalibration to be supported."
— Dr. Deilen Michelle Villegas

Functional & Holistic Approaches to Menopausal Support

These evidence-informed tools help restore balance, protect bone and cardiovascular health, and ease emotional and physiological symptoms—without overriding the body's natural process.

1. Phytoestrogens: Nature's Gentle Estrogen Modulators

Phytoestrogens are plant compounds that weakly bind to estrogen receptors in the body. While their action is far milder than endogenous estrogen or HRT, they can help buffer the dramatic fluctuations of menopause.

- **Flaxseeds** – Rich in lignans, shown to support estrogen metabolism and reduce hot flashes

- **Soy (non-GMO, fermented)** – Contains isoflavones that modulate estrogen activity; beneficial for bone density and vasomotor symptoms

- **Red clover** – Contains bioavailable isoflavones, shown to reduce frequency/severity of hot flashes in some women

These foods act as **modulators**, not hormones, helping the body gently adapt rather than forcing it into a specific state.

2. Adaptogens: Rewiring the Stress-Hormone Loop

Adaptogenic herbs help recalibrate the hypothalamic-pituitary-adrenal (HPA) axis, which becomes **hyperactive during menopause** due to decreased ovarian output and increased reliance on adrenal hormone production.

- **Ashwagandha** – Supports adrenal resilience, reduces anxiety, and promotes sleep

- **Rhodiola** – Enhances energy, combats fatigue, and improves cognitive clarity

- **Shatavari** – A traditional Ayurvedic herb revered for balancing female hormones, soothing dryness, and enhancing libido

Adaptogens don't just manage stress—they **restore the body's capacity to respond** to it in harmony.

3. Foundational Nutrients for Hormonal Harmony

Menopause increases the demand for specific nutrients that support bone health, mood regulation, cardiovascular protection, and hormonal detoxification.

- **Magnesium glycinate or citrate** – Supports sleep, reduces anxiety, and eases muscle tension

- **Vitamin D3 + K2** – Vital for bone density, immune function, and hormonal balance

- **Omega-3 fatty acids (EPA/DHA)** – Reduce inflammation, support brain health, and stabilize mood

- **B-complex vitamins** – Support methylation, energy, and neurotransmitter synthesis

These micronutrients act as the **building blocks for biochemical transformation** during this sacred life shift.

4. Mindfulness, Nervous System Regulation & Sleep Rituals

Hormonal changes affect the limbic system, circadian rhythms, and cortisol response—often manifesting as **emotional reactivity, insomnia, and anxiety.** Rather than numbing these symptoms, we must support the body's recalibration with **nervous system nourishment**.

- **Breathwork and meditation** – Calm the amygdala and enhance parasympathetic tone

- **Sleep hygiene rituals** – Dim lighting, magnesium baths, blue light blockers, chamomile or valerian teas

- **Somatic movement** – Restorative yoga, tai chi, walking, or dancing to reconnect with the body

- **Therapeutic journaling** – To process identity shifts and track patterns of emotional and physical change

Menopause asks us to **slow down and listen**—not just to our symptoms, but to the deeper stories our bodies are trying to tell.

Clinical Guidance & Caution

While HRT can be a valuable tool—especially in cases of early menopause, severe osteoporosis risk, or premature ovarian insufficiency—it should be **individualized and closely monitored**. Practitioners should assess:

- Hormone levels (via DUTCH test or serum labs)

- Cardiovascular and cancer risk history

- Lifestyle and psycho-spiritual readiness for alternative therapies

An integrative protocol might include **low-dose HRT supported by phytonutrients, detox pathways, and nervous system practices**, offering the best of both worlds when needed.

> "Menopause is not a condition to manage—it is a transition to honor. The goal is not to erase the changes, but to **move through them with grace, tools, and truth**."
> — Dr. Villegas

By offering women comprehensive, respectful, and personalized care—whether through HRT, herbs, nutrition, or spiritual ritual—we move away from a model of suppression and into one of **sovereignty and embodiment**.

Visual: Menopause as Transformation Chart

Phase	Common Experience	Holistic Support
Perimenopause	Mood swings,	Hormone testing, adaptogens,

	irregular cycles	nervous system care
Menopause	Hot flashes, sleep changes, libido	Phytoestrogens, mindfulness, strength training
Postmenopause	Emotional rebirth, energy shifts	Creativity, spiritual practice, community

Cultural Wisdom & Menopausal Archetypes

In many Indigenous, African, Eastern, and Earth-honoring traditions, **menopause was never pathologized—it was revered.** It was not seen as a loss, but as a sacred transition into one's **deepest power.** While modern Western medicine frames menopause as an "end" or "decline," our ancestral lineages recognized it as a **spiritual ascension**—a second birth into a new archetype: the Crone, the Wisdom-Keeper, the Medicine Woman, the Elder.

> "In cultures that remember their roots, menopausal women don't disappear—they *emerge*."
> — Dr. Deilen Michelle Villegas

The Crone: Keeper of Wise Blood

The word *Crone*, often used as a slur in modern society, originally meant "crowned one." She is not the withered woman of cultural caricature, but the **sovereign** one—crowned with experience, insight, and authority. Her blood no longer flows outward, but is retained as *wise blood*, circulating inward, intensifying her intuitive gifts and energetic presence.

In ancestral frameworks:

- **She was the midwife of death and rebirth**, guiding souls in transition—not just into the world, but out of it.

- **She held the medicine songs**, the root knowledge, the stories of the earth.

- **She sat in council**, offering the clarity of someone no longer clouded by external validation or hormonal cycles.

Menopause was seen as the **culmination of the feminine path**, not its decay. It was a moment when physical fertility gave way to **energetic and spiritual fertility.**

Global Traditions of Menopausal Reverence

✦ Indigenous African Traditions

In many African communities, elder women were seen as **spiritual intermediaries**, called upon for rituals, conflict resolution, and divination. Their dreams were considered sacred. Their bodies, no longer pulled by cycles, were viewed as *permanent temples*—stable, rooted, and potent.

✦ Native American Teachings

Some tribes taught that once a woman entered menopause, she had direct access to the Great Spirit. She was no longer "moontime-bound," meaning her energetic body was now a **living altar**, able to offer wisdom without interference. She became the teacher, the truth-speaker, the one who could walk between worlds.

✦ East Asian Philosophies

In Traditional Chinese Medicine, menopause is a transition from the reproductive phase (yang) to the **shen** phase— the spirit-centered time. Qi (life force) returns to the heart and brain, heightening intuition and spiritual insight. The woman becomes a guide, not just for her family, but for her community.

✦ Andean and Mesoamerican Cultures

Menopausal women in Andean traditions were referred to as **Abuelas Sabias**—Wise Grandmothers. They carried the medicine of plants, prayer, and prophecy. In Mesoamerican mythology, the Crone archetype was aligned with the **Owl Goddess**, a guardian of the night and the subconscious.

Reclaiming the Crone in Modern Times

In a world that fears aging and silences women beyond reproductive years, **reclaiming the menopausal archetype is an act of resistance and remembrance**. It is a cultural healing. It is a call back to the root.

Ways to honor and embody this sacred transition:

- **Ceremonial Rites**: Host a *Second Blood Ceremony* to honor the last bleed and welcome the wise years with ritual and reverence.

- **Storytelling Circles**: Gather with other women to share birth stories, love stories, grief, dreams, and ancestral memories. Menopause is a threshold—crossing it deserves witness.

- **Moon Rituals**: Even without bleeding, your body remains cyclical. Align with the moon to chart emotions, energy, and spiritual insight.

- **Elder Council Creation**: Form groups of women in their post-menopausal years to offer mentorship, healing, and cultural wisdom to younger generations.

- **Sacred Symbols**: Wear the spiral, the owl, or ancestral beads as symbols of your transition. Embody your eldership with pride and beauty.

"In reclaiming the Crone, we reclaim the rhythm of life. We restore the sacred seat of female eldership. We remember that our wisdom is not wasted—it is needed now more than ever."

— Dr. Deilen Michelle Villegas

Menopause is not just a biological process. It is a **spiritual initiation** that has been forgotten—but not lost. When we **revive the archetypes**, reawaken the ceremonies, and reclaim the stories of our elders, we restore the rightful power of the feminine at every stage of life.

Becoming the Firekeeper

Menopause is not a depletion—it is a *distillation*. It is the refinement of a woman's essence, not the loss of it. The fire that once burned to nourish others, create life, and maintain outward responsibilities does not go out—it burns cleaner, brighter, and with greater precision. What once flowed outward through blood, emotion, and duty now **returns to the center**—fueling intuition, creativity, and the fierce clarity of a woman who no longer needs permission to take up space.

> "The bleeding stops, but the birthing doesn't. Now you birth wisdom, discernment, and legacy."
> — Dr. Deilen Michelle Villegas

The Firekeeper Archetype

In many earth-based traditions, the Firekeeper was the one who watched over the sacred flames. Not just for warmth or light, but for memory—for ritual, for vision, for the continuation of stories and soul. She was the one who stayed awake while others slept, tending the hearth, singing to the embers, protecting what was holy and true.

The menopausal woman becomes the modern Firekeeper.

She no longer leaks her energy into every demand. She no longer fears being misunderstood. She no longer sacrifices her truth for belonging. Instead, she becomes:

- **The Truth-Teller**, even when her voice shakes

- **The Healer**, whose medicine is presence, perspective, and power

- **The Ancestral Bridge**, carrying memory forward while dreaming new futures

- **The Visionary**, who sees not with her eyes, but with her bones

From Fertility to Fervor

Where the fertile years once demanded softness and selflessness, the Firekeeper phase demands **ferocity and focus**. This is not the time for shrinking. It is the time for sharpening. For gathering the broken pieces of self and throwing them into the sacred fire—not to destroy them, but to *alchemize* them.

> "Menopause is your invitation to stop being everything for everyone and become who you were always meant to be."

This transition births:

- **Boundaries without guilt**

- **Desire without apology**

- **Vision without dilution**

The energy that once created children, built families, and held communities now becomes available for your own becoming.

Living from the Inner Flame

To become the Firekeeper is to **reclaim the flame within**. No longer governed by external cycles, your energy becomes sovereign. You no longer bleed, but you blaze. And that blaze can be directed anywhere—into activism, artistry, mentorship, healing, writing, leadership, spiritual work, or ancestral reclamation.

This fire is not chaotic—it is calibrated. It is the fire that cooks medicine. The fire that lights sacred ceremonies. The fire that clears the old to make room for the true.

Honoring This Sacred Role

In your practice, encourage women in this stage to:

- **Create a sacred hearth altar**: Adorned with candles, ancestral items, and symbols of fire

- **Revisit their life story**: What parts are ready to be released to the flames? What truths are rising from the ashes?

- **Initiate a Firekeeper Ceremony**: Invite sisters, mentors, or even self-guided rituals to mark the transition from fertility to fiery sovereignty

- **Identify their legacy work**: What are you here to preserve, teach, birth, or dismantle?

"The fire within you was never meant to dim with age—it was meant to become eternal."

— Dr. Deilen Michelle Villegas

References

Greendale, G. A., & Gold, E. B. (2005). Lifestyle factors: Are they related to vasomotor symptoms and menopause? *Menopause, 12*(6), 777–784. https://doi.org/10.1097/01.gme.0000185263.33314.49

North American Menopause Society. (2022). *Menopause practice: A clinician's guide*. https://www.menopause.org/docs/default-source/professional/nams-clinician%E2%80%99s-guide-to-menopause-practice

Taylor, M. (2001). Alternative medicine and the perimenopause. *Clinical Obstetrics and Gynecology, 44*(4), 774–785. https://doi.org/10.1097/00003081-200112000-00019

CHAPTER 9

Profiling Hypo-Function in Males

The Silent Shift

Male hormonal decline does not arrive with a warning bell. There are no sudden stoppages, no celebratory ceremonies, no culturally supported transitions. Instead, it creeps in like a shadow—gradual, invisible, and often mistaken for stress, aging, or lack of willpower. This decline in testosterone and other androgens, known as **andropause**, **late-onset hypogonadism**, or **male hypo-function**, is real and significant —but frequently missed in clinical settings and even more so in everyday conversations.

Unlike menopause, which often comes with unmistakable symptoms and public acknowledgment, **andropause is silent and stigmatized**. Men may begin to experience changes as early as their 30s, yet go untreated for decades—if they're ever treated at all.

> "Masculinity is not lost with testosterone—it is redefined with awareness."
> — Dr. Deilen Michelle Villegas

Understanding Male Hypo-Function

Testosterone, the primary male sex hormone, is crucial not just for sexual performance, but for **energy levels, mental clarity, emotional stability, muscle mass, motivation, and even spiritual drive**. It interacts with other hormones like DHEA, estradiol, cortisol, and thyroid hormones—creating a complex endocrine network that governs physical and emotional vitality.

Common Symptoms of Andropause:

- Declining libido or erectile function

- Muscle weakness and increased abdominal fat

- Brain fog, low motivation, and difficulty concentrating

- Mood changes: depression, irritability, emotional flatness

- Sleep disturbances and reduced recovery from exercise

- Feelings of inadequacy, isolation, or spiritual disconnection

What makes andropause particularly insidious is that these symptoms are often **rationalized away**—blamed on aging, burnout, or midlife crisis. In truth, they may reflect a deep physiological shift that requires both clinical and holistic attention.

The Psychological Impact of Unspoken Decline

In cultures that define manhood through performance, productivity, and potency, admitting to fatigue, emotional shifts, or sexual dysfunction can feel like failure. This silence becomes a form of suffering.

Men often internalize the belief that seeking help is weakness. Instead of asking for hormonal testing or emotional support, they may withdraw, become irritable, overcompensate with risk-taking, or spiral into depression.

Andropause isn't just a biological event—it's an identity crisis in disguise.

A Cultural Call to Redefine Masculinity

We need a new narrative. One that reframes hormonal changes not as emasculating, but as **evolutionary**. As testosterone declines, the body is not betraying the man—it's inviting him into **a new stage of wisdom, presence, and inner mastery.**

The "warrior" archetype gives way to the **sage**—the man whose power is no longer measured by dominance, but by discernment.

Root Causes Beyond Aging

While aging is natural, **accelerated hypo-function is not**. The modern man is facing unprecedented hormonal disruption due to:

- **Chronic stress and elevated cortisol**, which suppresses testosterone

- **Endocrine disruptors** like BPA, phthalates, and heavy metals

- **Poor sleep quality**, which impairs testosterone regeneration (most of which is produced during REM sleep)

- **Nutrient depletion**, especially of zinc, magnesium, B vitamins, and essential fats

- **Alcohol, medications, and inflammatory diets** that tax the liver and hormonal pathways

In truth, much of what is labeled as "just getting older" is actually **preventable or reversible dysfunction**—when addressed with an integrative lens.

The Holistic Healing Invitation

Supporting men through this transition requires more than testosterone therapy. It requires a **soul-centered, body-informed approach** that includes:

- **Hormonal Testing**: Free and total testosterone, DHEA, cortisol, estradiol, SHBG, LH/FSH, thyroid function

- **Lifestyle Optimization**: Strength training, sleep hygiene, sunlight exposure, stress resilience training

- **Functional Nutrition**: High-quality proteins, healthy fats, adaptogens like ashwagandha and tongkat ali

- **Emotional Integration**: Therapy, men's groups, rites of passage, and deep inner work

- **Sexual Reclamation**: Mindful intimacy, somatic work, and redefining sex beyond performance

"There is a season for initiation in every man's life. Andropause is not the end of virility—it is the beginning of embodied masculinity."

Younger Men and Hormonal Burnout: A Rising Concern

While andropause has historically been associated with middle-aged men, an alarming trend is emerging—**increasing numbers of men in their 20s and early 30s are showing signs of hormonal hypo-function**. Fatigue. Loss of libido. Emotional flatness. Brain fog. Erectile difficulties. These are no longer symptoms reserved for aging—they are the red flags of a generation under siege.

And nowhere is this crisis more pronounced than in **Black, Indigenous, and communities of color**, where systemic oppression compounds biological stressors. When we add up the pressures of racial trauma, environmental toxins, medical neglect, and socio-economic barriers, we find a hormonal crisis masquerading as laziness, low drive, or "mental health issues." But the truth is, **these young men are burnt out before they've even had the chance to fully embody their masculine**

potential.

> "Hormonal collapse in young men is not weakness —it is the body's protest against unsustainable survival."
> — Dr. Deilen Michelle Villegas

Key Drivers in Younger Men

1. Chronic Nervous System Dysregulation

In the face of intergenerational trauma, societal hypervigilance, and ongoing racialized stress, the nervous system stays trapped in **sympathetic overdrive**. This constant activation of the **hypothalamic-pituitary-adrenal (HPA) axis** floods the body with cortisol, which in turn **suppresses testosterone**, disrupts dopamine function, and erodes resilience.

Symptoms may present as:

- Emotional numbness or irritability

- Sleep disturbances and intrusive thoughts

- Avoidant behaviors and substance coping

- Disconnection from purpose and drive

This is **not apathy**—it's adrenal depletion.

2. Drug Use and Misuse

The normalization of substance use in modern culture— especially within overworked and underserved populations— has a direct effect on hormone health:

- **Opioids** inhibit the release of gonadotropin-releasing hormone (GnRH), reducing testosterone production

- **Cannabis**, when overused, has been shown to reduce sperm count and disrupt testosterone levels

- **Stimulants** like Adderall and cocaine spike cortisol, disrupt sleep cycles, and lead to burnout

- **ED drugs** like sildenafil (Viagra), when used recreationally, can **create psychological dependence and suppress natural arousal pathways**

These substances offer short-term relief but often leave young men hormonally hijacked in the long run.

3. Porn-Induced Erectile Dysfunction (PIED)

In the age of unlimited digital access, many young men are **exposed to high-dopamine sexual content before they even engage in real-life intimacy**. The result? A generation that is overstimulated but under-connected.

PIED is driven by:

- **Dopamine desensitization**: leading to lack of arousal with real partners

- **Performance anxiety** and shame-based self-worth

- **Emotional detachment** from sex as a bonding or sacred act

This form of sexual dysfunction is not rooted in physiology —but in the **disruption of the brain's reward system**. And unless addressed through detox, somatic reintegration, and sexual re-education, it can have long-term consequences on relationships, fertility, and self-identity.

4. Poor Diet and Sedentary Lifestyle

Food is information, and modern diets are sending the wrong signals. The **standard American diet (SAD)**—high in refined sugar, inflammatory oils, and ultra-processed junk—contributes to:

- **Insulin resistance**: which increases estrogen and suppresses testosterone

- **Visceral fat accumulation**: especially around the abdomen, where fat cells convert testosterone into estrogen via aromatase

- **Gut inflammation**: impairing nutrient absorption critical for hormone synthesis (e.g., zinc, B6, magnesium)

Coupled with sedentary living, screen fatigue, and lack of sunlight, this lifestyle **shuts down the body's natural testosterone production and energetic expression.**

A Generation at a Crossroads

When you put these drivers together, you get a devastating equation: **Young men are losing their hormonal resilience before they even get a chance to fully harness it.**

But this isn't about returning to outdated models of masculinity. This is about **restoring vitality, honoring vulnerability, and reclaiming embodiment**. We must teach young men that strength isn't just physical—it's **nervous system sovereignty**, **sexual self-awareness**, and **emotional literacy.**

The Road to Recovery Must Be Holistic

Supporting this generation of men requires more than lab tests and prescriptions. It demands a **multidimensional response:**

- **Hormone Panels**: Assess total and free testosterone, cortisol, SHBG, prolactin, and DHEA

- **Nervous System Healing**: Breathwork, vagus nerve toning, trauma-informed therapy

- **Nutritional Repair**: Whole foods, elimination of endocrine disruptors, gut restoration protocols

- **Digital Detox**: Reducing screen time, social media comparison, and pornography exposure

- **Purpose Activation**: Helping men reconnect to mission, movement, and meaning

> "We must stop pathologizing young men's exhaustion and start treating the systems that are depleting them."

Case Study: Isaiah's Recovery

Isaiah, a 28-year-old Latino client, came to counseling reporting fatigue, depression, and loss of sexual interest. He was using marijuana daily, spent hours watching pornography, and worked night shifts with poor sleep hygiene. Labs showed borderline low testosterone and elevated cortisol.

An integrative plan included:

- Trauma-informed somatic therapy and EMDR to address early childhood stress
- Gradual reduction of cannabis and complete break from pornography
- Strength training, sleep cycle regulation, and B-complex with zinc
- Nervous system regulation through breathwork,

meditation, and adaptogens

After five months, Isaiah reported improved erections, reduced anxiety, and greater emotional presence in his relationship.

Case Study: Malcolm's Reckoning

Malcolm, a 45-year-old African American father of two, arrived in counseling feeling "numb and exhausted." Once a competitive athlete, he now struggled with depression, weight gain, and low libido. Lab results showed:

- Total testosterone: 320 ng/dL (low-normal)
- SHBG: Elevated
- Estradiol: Elevated

His protocol included:

- Resistance training and interval cardio 3x/week
- Zinc and DIM supplementation to support testosterone metabolism
- Sleep optimization through blue light blocking and magnesium
- Couples therapy to address emotional disconnection

By month four, Malcolm's energy improved, his libido returned, and he described feeling "awake for the first time in years."

The SHBG Connection

Sex Hormone-Binding Globulin (SHBG) is one of the least talked about yet most influential regulators of male hormone health. Produced primarily in the liver, SHBG acts as a transport protein—it binds tightly to sex hormones like testosterone and estrogen, escorting them through the bloodstream. But here's the catch: **once testosterone is bound to SHBG, it becomes biologically inactive.** Only **free testosterone**—the unbound fraction—is available to exert its effects on libido, mood, muscle mass, motivation, and metabolic function.

In essence, **SHBG is the gatekeeper of male vitality**. When levels are too high, even men with "normal" total testosterone may experience the full spectrum of low-T symptoms: fatigue, erectile difficulties, low drive, and brain fog. And yet, SHBG is rarely discussed in conventional hormone panels, leaving many men misdiagnosed or overlooked.

What Causes Elevated SHBG?

Elevated SHBG isn't random—it is often the body's adaptation to stress, inflammation, or endocrine imbalance. Key contributors include:

- **Aging**: SHBG naturally increases with age, especially after 40

- **Liver Dysfunction**: The liver regulates SHBG production; chronic alcohol use, fatty liver, or inflammation can skew levels

- **Thyroid Imbalance**: Hyperthyroidism increases SHBG, while hypothyroidism decreases it

- **High Estrogen Levels**: Aromatization of testosterone into estrogen (common in abdominal fat) raises SHBG

- **Nutritional Deficiencies**: Low zinc, protein, and vitamin D can impair SHBG regulation

- **Insulin Sensitivity**: Paradoxically, insulin resistance **lowers** SHBG (increasing free testosterone), but at the cost of inflammation and androgen dominance

So while elevated SHBG may appear protective on paper, it can quietly **strip a man of his access to vitality** by locking away the very hormone that fuels drive, power, and presence.

Lab Interpretation: Go Beyond the Surface

Total testosterone is not the full story. A man can have "normal" total testosterone but still suffer from symptoms of hormonal depletion due to high SHBG.

Request a Full Hormone Panel that includes:

- Total Testosterone

- **Free Testosterone** (calculated or direct)

- SHBG

- Estradiol (E2)

- DHEA-S

- Albumin

- TSH, Free T3, Free T4 (thyroid markers)

- Liver enzymes (ALT, AST, GGT)

This full-spectrum view gives practitioners insight into whether testosterone is **available** and **usable**, not just floating around bound and dormant.

Functional Strategies for Lowering SHBG & Reclaiming Testosterone

Healing male hormone health isn't about "hacking" masculinity—it's about restoring biological safety and energetic flow. These holistic interventions help optimize SHBG and unlock free testosterone:

1. Adaptogenic Herbs

- **Ashwagandha**: Lowers cortisol, enhances testosterone, improves sperm quality

- **Tongkat Ali**: Shown in clinical trials to increase free testosterone and reduce SHBG

- **Panax Ginseng**: Improves erectile function, vitality, and stress resilience

  These botanicals act as endocrine allies—supporting the body's hormonal harmony rather than overriding it.

2. Nutritional Therapy

- **High-protein diets** help regulate SHBG and support liver detox pathways

- **Healthy fats** (avocados, olive oil, nuts, pasture-raised meats) are precursors for hormone production

- **Cruciferous vegetables** (broccoli, cauliflower, arugula) assist in estrogen metabolism and reduce aromatization

- **Zinc and Vitamin D** support androgen function and SHBG modulation

Think of food not as fuel—but as **messengers that rewire your endocrine system**.

3. Strength Training & Movement

- **Resistance training** (especially heavy compound lifts) increases free testosterone and downregulates SHBG

- **HIIT and sprints** support insulin sensitivity and metabolic resilience

- **Daily movement** improves lymphatic flow, mitochondrial efficiency, and mood stabilization

Movement is not just physical—it's **energetic reclamation.**

4. Mitochondrial Therapies: Cold and Heat

- **Cold exposure** (ice baths, cold showers) boosts testosterone and norepinephrine

- **Sauna therapy** enhances detoxification, reduces stress load, and supports natural hormone rhythms

- Both cold and heat improve **mitochondrial function**, the powerhouses that drive cellular energy, fertility, and hormone signaling

These ancestral tools teach the nervous system how to adapt, **harness stress wisely**, and rebalance hormonal output.

Awareness as Power

Elevated SHBG is not just a lab anomaly—it's a reflection of the body's adaptive intelligence in response to stress, toxicity, or stagnation. When we begin to track these markers and implement functional solutions, we don't just raise testosterone—we **restore a man's vitality, clarity, and embodied leadership.**

> "Masculinity is not manufactured in a supplement bottle. It is cultivated through awareness, nourishment, and radical self-responsibility."
> — Dr. Deilen Michelle Villegas

Emotional Impacts of Hormonal Decline

"When a man no longer feels his fire, he may question if he is still a

flame." – Dr. Deilen Michelle Villegas

Male hormonal hypo-function doesn't just affect the body—it strikes at the very root of identity, purpose, and emotional resilience. As testosterone wanes, libido slows, energy dips, and focus blurs, many men report a gnawing disconnection from who they once were. The change is subtle at first—fatigue here, irritability there—but over time, it can erode confidence, ambition, and intimate connection.

The Crisis of Masculine Identity

In a culture that ties masculinity to performance—sexual prowess, physical strength, productivity, and stoicism—hormonal decline can feel like personal failure. Without guidance or language to articulate these internal shifts, men often retreat into shame, secrecy, or self-sabotage.

This quiet unraveling may show up as:

- Emotional withdrawal from partners or children

- Heightened reactivity or frustration

- Obsessive exercise or overwork to "feel capable again"

- Substance use or risky behaviors to artificially stimulate dopamine

- Avoidance of intimacy due to fear of inadequacy

And yet, beneath these behaviors is not weakness—but **unprocessed grief** for the version of self that no longer fits. What men often need is not more pressure to "perform," but space to evolve into a more conscious embodiment of manhood.

Hormones and Emotional Resilience

Testosterone and DHEA don't just fuel muscle mass—they **regulate neurotransmitters** like dopamine and serotonin. This is why low testosterone is often mistaken for depression or anxiety. A man may not be "mentally ill"—he may be hormonally depleted, unbalanced, and spiritually disoriented.

Common emotional experiences associated with male hypo-function:

- Low self-esteem or imposter syndrome

- Reduced motivation, focus, and drive

- Difficulty experiencing joy or connection

- Emotional numbness or apathy

- Disorientation around purpose and future goals

Left unaddressed, these symptoms can manifest as midlife crisis, infidelity, financial recklessness, or emotional collapse.

Therapeutic Interventions Must Evolve

Addressing the emotional impact of hormonal decline requires a trauma-informed, nervous system-aware approach. Men must be given tools that don't just restore their hormones —but **reframe their identity** beyond the outdated metrics of performance.

1. Emotional Literacy and Somatic Therapy

- Teach men how to **name and normalize their inner states**

- Use somatic practices to help them **feel safe in their own body** again

- Address grief, anger, and shame as valid emotional responses—not weaknesses

- Reconnect breath with presence, and sensation with truth

Many men haven't shut down their emotions—they were never taught how to stay present with them.

2. Education on Hormonal Shifts

- Demystify the science of andropause

- Normalize emotional fluctuations and libido changes as part of midlife recalibration

- Encourage regular hormone panels as part of holistic health, not crisis response

- Provide clarity that masculinity evolves—it doesn't disappear

Men need **data, validation, and nonjudgmental space** to integrate this phase.

3. Redefining Masculinity as Relational, Not Just Performative

- Challenge the narrative that a man's worth is tied to erections, income, or intensity

- Uplift values of **presence, emotional availability, and energetic integrity**

- Support healthy interdependence, vulnerability, and emotional leadership

- Celebrate men for their depth, not just their output

Mature masculinity is not about domination—it's about devotion to something greater than ego.

4. Reconnection with Body and Spirit

- Introduce mindful movement, breathwork, and embodiment practices

- Offer nature immersion, rites of passage, or ancestral ritual as initiation into elderhood

- Use sexuality as a space for self-discovery and soul connection—not just performance

- Invite spiritual mentorship, community dialogue, or sacred brotherhood circles

When men reclaim their emotional and spiritual selves, **a deeper version of power emerges**—one rooted not in dominance, but in conscious presence and embodied wisdom.

The hormonal shift in men is not a curse—it's a **call to awakening**. It asks men to slow down, turn inward, and redefine strength not as how much they can carry, but how deeply they can feel. When this transition is honored rather than hidden, it becomes an initiation into a new kind of leadership—rooted in balance, awareness, and self-possession.

"A man does not become less by feeling more. He becomes whole." – Dr. Deilen Michelle Villegas

Visual: Male Hormone Decline TimelineRedefining Vitality

Age Range	Typical Hormonal Trends	Support Strategies
20–30	Burnout from stress, trauma, substances	Nervous system regulation, trauma

		healing
30–40	Slow testosterone decline begins	Stress management, sleep, exercise
40–55	SHBG rises, libido and energy wane	Hormone testing, adaptogens, therapy
55+	DHEA/testosterone drop significantly	Anti-inflammatory nutrition, emotional care

"Vitality is not lost—it evolves. And in that evolution, there is power." – Dr. Deilen Michelle Villegas

Hormonal decline is not a moral failing, nor a sign of broken masculinity. It is a **biological reality**—one that every man will encounter, yet few are prepared to navigate. In truth, this shift offers not an ending, but a **threshold**. A powerful turning point where the definition of strength must be reclaimed, redefined, and expanded.

Vitality Beyond Testosterone

Vitality has long been measured by physical prowess, sexual frequency, and adrenaline-fueled performance. But true vitality is not measured by how fast a man moves—it is reflected in **how deeply he is rooted in himself**.

Hormonal hypo-function does not erase a man's power. Rather, it **redirects it inward**—toward reflection, relational depth, spiritual attunement, and legacy-building. The physical decline becomes a metaphorical descent into self-inquiry. And when honored, it births a more conscious masculinity, unburdened by ego and driven by embodiment.

From Performance to Presence

As testosterone naturally wanes, men are invited to shed the performative shells of youth—the constant striving, the need to conquer, the fear of emotional vulnerability. What remains is not emptiness, but **essence**.

This stage of life asks:

- Can you show up fully, even when your energy shifts?

- Can you honor your emotional truth without shame?

- Can you explore intimacy through presence, not pressure?

- Can you redefine your worth beyond productivity?

This is not about giving up—it's about **growing up**. And in that growth, there is the possibility of deeper joy, truer love, and more meaningful connection with self and others.

Holistic Pathways to Sustainable Energy

Redefining vitality also means tending to the terrain: the nervous system, metabolism, mitochondria, and emotional landscape that fuel sustainable wellness.

Functional strategies for lasting vitality include:

- **Regenerative movement**: strength training, qigong, walking meditations

- **Hormone-balancing nutrition**: zinc, magnesium, cruciferous vegetables, omega-3s

- **Mitochondrial support**: CoQ10, NAD+, sauna, cold exposure

- **Emotional hygiene**: journaling, therapy, breathwork, meaningful conversations

- **Spiritual anchoring**: meditation, ancestral practice, time in nature

Vitality, in this phase, is about **rhythm over rush, depth over domination, connection over conquest.**

The New Face of Male Leadership

When men honor the inner changes of andropause with curiosity and care, they unlock a version of masculinity that this world desperately needs—**heart-centered, embodied, emotionally attuned, and wise.**

This version of manhood doesn't chase youth—it **cultivates legacy.**
It doesn't suppress change—it **integrates it into purpose.**
It doesn't fear decline—it **transforms it into devotion.**

> "Hormonal decline is not the end of a man's vitality. It is the beginning of his sovereignty." – Dr. Deilen Michelle Villegas

References

Basaria, S., & Dobs, A. S. (2001). Hypogonadism and androgen replacement therapy in elderly men. *American Journal of Medicine, 110*(7), 563–572. https://doi.org/10.1016/S0002-9343(01)00641-7

Morgentaler, A., & Traish, A. M. (2009). Shifting the paradigm of testosterone and prostate cancer: The saturation model and the limits of androgen-dependent growth. *European Urology, 55*(2), 310–320. https://doi.org/10.1016/j.eururo.2008.09.024

Zitzmann, M. (2006). Testosterone deficiency, insulin resistance and the metabolic syndrome. *Nature Clinical Practice Urology, 3*(12), 621–628. https://doi.org/10.1038/ncpuro0639

CHAPTER 10

Male Pattern Hair Loss & What It Reveals

Hair is more than protein strands—it's an intimate thread in the story of **self-perception**, **status**, and **sexual identity**. In nearly every culture, a man's hair has carried unspoken messages: youth, virility, dominance, desirability, and even leadership. When it begins to fall, the loss is rarely just physical —it becomes **a psychic unraveling**, silently challenging a man's sense of worth, power, and aging.

Male pattern hair loss (MPHL), also known as androgenetic alopecia, affects nearly 50% of men by age 50 (Norwood, 1975). But while it's often dismissed as a cosmetic concern or an inevitable genetic trait, the reality is far more layered. Hair loss can be a **clinical symptom of internal imbalance**, a **psychological trigger**, and a **spiritual threshold**—a portal into deeper questions of identity, purpose, and perception.

Beneath the Surface: Biology and Beyond

MPHL is primarily driven by the conversion of testosterone into **dihydrotestosterone (DHT)**—a more potent androgen that binds to scalp hair follicles, miniaturizing them and shortening the hair growth cycle. However, this biochemical pathway does not occur in a vacuum.

Contributing factors include:

- **High cortisol and chronic stress**, which accelerate inflammation and hormonal conversion

- **Poor liver detoxification**, which reduces the body's ability to metabolize DHT and estrogens

- **Nutrient deficiencies** (zinc, biotin, iron, vitamin D, B-complex) that impair follicle strength and resilience

- **Inflammatory diets** rich in sugar and seed oils that fuel oxidative stress

- **Thyroid dysfunction** or autoimmune triggers like Hashimoto's, which may contribute to diffuse or patchy hair loss

Thus, hair loss becomes an outer **mirror of inner dysregulation**.

Hair Loss and the Male Psyche

For many men, the shedding of hair is experienced as the shedding of identity. Society rarely prepares them to grieve this loss. Instead, they are expected to laugh it off, shave it down, or mask it with prescriptions.

But beneath the cultural humor lies quiet pain:

- A fear of **no longer being attractive or desired**

- A sense of **losing youth, status, or competitiveness**

- Anxiety around **career visibility or romantic rejection**

- Even existential dread—**"If I am no longer virile, who am I?"**

In therapy and clinical work, these themes often emerge not in the form of "I'm upset about my hair," but in a man's unspoken withdrawal from intimacy, reluctance to be seen, or diminished confidence in leadership roles.

> *"Hair loss can activate shame—but it can also awaken sovereignty. The power lies in what meaning you choose*

to assign it." – Dr. Deilen Michelle Villegas

Holistic Strategies for Root-Level Healing

While some men opt for medications like finasteride or minoxidil, many experience side effects such as sexual dysfunction or mood changes. A root-cause, integrative approach focuses on restoring the inner terrain—not just manipulating symptoms.

Foundational protocols may include:

- **DHT modulation**: Saw palmetto, nettle root, pumpkin seed oil, spearmint tea

- **Liver support**: Milk thistle, dandelion, NAC, castor oil packs

- **Micronutrient repletion**: Iron, zinc, silica, collagen, B-complex, vitamin D3

- **Stress regulation**: Adaptogens like ashwagandha and reishi, breathwork, nervous system tracking

- **Scalp health**: Rosemary oil, scalp massage, red light therapy, microneedling

- **Thyroid and gut testing** to rule out deeper endocrine or autoimmune contributors

And perhaps most importantly—**addressing the emotional narrative** that has become entangled with the hair.

The Sacred Reframe: Reclaiming the Crown

Hair loss does not define a man's masculinity. **Presence, integrity, emotional depth, and inner leadership** do.

Some men emerge from the experience of hair loss with deeper embodiment, having shed false attachments to external validation. Others reclaim their power through rituals of shaving, styling, or adorning the scalp with confidence and pride. Either path, when chosen consciously, can be a rite of passage into **sovereign self-expression.**

Let this chapter serve not as a prescription—but an invitation:

- To heal the root.

- To honor the grief.

- To rewrite the story of what it means to be powerful, even as the crown changes form.

DHT, Nutrient Deficiency, and Genetic Sensitivity: The Triad of Hair Loss

At the core of male pattern hair loss (MPHL) lies a biochemical process that has long been oversimplified. The conversion of testosterone into **dihydrotestosterone (DHT)** via the enzyme **5-alpha-reductase** is a well-documented mechanism. Elevated DHT levels bind to androgen receptors in scalp hair follicles—particularly along the crown and temples—leading to **miniaturization** of follicles, a shortened growth (anagen) phase, and eventual hair thinning (Randall, 2008).

But the real story is more nuanced. DHT is not inherently "bad." It plays a vital role in libido, bone density, and male development. The problem lies in the **context in which DHT becomes dysregulated**—a terrain shaped by nutritional status, stress, detoxification capacity, and genetic expression.

Beyond DHT: The Nutritional and Genetic Landscape

Hair is a metabolically active tissue that relies on consistent nutrient supply and cellular signaling. Deficiencies in key micronutrients can make the follicles more vulnerable to the effects of DHT—**amplifying its impact even at normal**

levels. This is where functional medicine and nutritional biochemistry offer clarity.

Common Nutritional Deficiencies Linked to Hair Loss:

- **Zinc**: A cofactor in over 300 enzymatic reactions, zinc is essential for follicle regeneration and DHT metabolism. Deficiency impairs testosterone balance and immune regulation within the scalp.

- **Vitamin D**: Plays a regulatory role in hair follicle cycling, immune modulation, and keratinocyte growth. Low levels are correlated with alopecia areata and MPHL.

- **Iron (Ferritin)**: Iron deficiency—particularly low ferritin levels—disrupts the transition of hair from the resting (telogen) to growth (anagen) phase. Even marginally low ferritin (<70 ng/mL) can impair hair growth.

- **Biotin**: A B-complex vitamin critical for keratin synthesis, scalp hydration, and the structural integrity of hair shafts. Often depleted by gut dysbiosis, antibiotics, and alcohol use.

Compounding these deficiencies, **chronic stress** increases cortisol levels, which can dysregulate the hypothalamic-pituitary-gonadal (HPG) axis. This indirectly raises 5-alpha-reductase activity, increasing DHT conversion while simultaneously **depleting the nutrients needed to buffer its effects**. This vicious cycle sets the stage for early and accelerated hair loss, even in younger men.

Genetic Sensitivity: Why Some Men Keep Their Hair

Not all men with high DHT levels experience hair loss—highlighting the role of **genetic polymorphisms**. Variations in the **androgen receptor (AR) gene**, particularly on the X chromosome, can make scalp follicles **more sensitive** to DHT's binding action (Ellis et al., 2001). Men with these polymorphisms are genetically predisposed to follicular miniaturization—even at "normal" androgen levels.

Other contributing genetic factors include:

- Variants in **SRD5A2** (the gene encoding 5-alpha-reductase)

- Genes involved in **inflammation and oxidative stress** (e.g., IL-6, TNF-alpha)

- Polymorphisms in **vitamin D receptor (VDR)** genes affecting follicle responsiveness

This explains why hair loss is **a bio-individual response**, not a universal male destiny.

> "DHT is a signal—but the body's terrain determines whether that signal harms or heals." – Dr. Deilen Michelle Villegas

Putting It Together: Root-Cause Integration

The key takeaway: **DHT is just one piece of the puzzle**. Nutrient depletion, systemic stress, toxic load, and genetic susceptibility converge to create the internal conditions that allow hair loss to progress.

An effective therapeutic approach includes:

- **Nutrient repletion**: personalized supplementation based on labs (zinc, ferritin, vitamin D, biotin)

- **Anti-DHT support**: natural 5-alpha-reductase inhibitors (saw palmetto, pumpkin seed oil, pygeum)

- **Stress modulation**: adaptogens, breathwork, nervous system tracking

- **Genetic testing** (if accessible) to assess AR gene sensitivity and methylation status

Chart: Relationship Between DHT, Nutrient Status, and Hair Loss Severity

Category	Mild Hair Loss	Moderate Hair Loss	Advanced Hair Loss
DHT Levels	Slightly elevated	Elevated	Significantly elevated
Zinc	Borderline low	Deficient	Severely deficient
Vitamin D	Within low-normal range	Deficient	Severely deficient
Iron (Ferritin)	Slightly depleted	Low	Critically low
Genetic Sensitivity	Minimal	Moderate	High
Psychological Impact	Mild insecurity	Social withdrawal	Low confidence, depression

Psychosexual Identity & Appearance: Reclaiming the Sacred Masculine

The loss of hair is more than a physical shift—it can mark a profound identity rupture. In many cultures, **hair is a symbol of virility, youth, vitality, and masculine prowess**. It is subconsciously linked to dominance, desirability, and power. So when a man begins to lose his hair, it often triggers a silent unraveling of his **psychosexual self-concept**.

This is not vanity—it is vulnerability.

From adolescence, many boys are conditioned to associate manhood with how they look, how they perform, and how they're perceived. Hair, muscles, height, and sexual stamina become the unspoken currencies of worth. When one of those attributes fades—like hair—it can feel like a loss of identity, even when sexual function itself remains intact.

Emotional Responses Often Seen in Clinical Practice:

- **Reduced sexual initiative** due to feelings of diminished attractiveness

- **Avoidance of intimacy or eye contact**, fearing rejection or invisibility

- **Hyperfixation on signs of aging**, leading to internalized shame or resentment

- **Withdrawal from social environments**, reinforcing isolation and lowered self-esteem

- **Self-objectification**—judging themselves through the imagined gaze of others

The pain is real—not just because of the mirror, but because of what society has projected onto that reflection.

The Neuropsychology of Appearance-Based Identity

Research in neuropsychology shows that **self-perception is deeply tied to body image**, especially when cultural scripts reinforce external validation. For men experiencing MPHL, this can result in:

- **Increased cortisol** from chronic shame or perceived rejection

- **Low dopamine** and reduced reward-seeking behavior (e.g., intimacy, goal pursuit)

- **Depressive symptoms**, including apathy, social fatigue, and loss of motivation

When a man's self-worth becomes entangled with a disappearing hairline, the internal landscape suffers. This isn't simply about aesthetics—it's about what the hair *represented* in terms of safety, belonging, and identity.

The Sacred Reframe: From Ego Image to Embodied Masculinity

What's often missing in public discourse and clinical care is the **sacred narrative**. Hair loss, when approached consciously, becomes more than a cosmetic concern—it becomes a **portal to emotional liberation** and an **invitation into spiritual maturity**.

> "A man's medicine doesn't live in his hair—it lives in his presence." – Dr. Deilen Michelle Villegas

This sacred masculine journey invites:

- **Decoupling worth from appearance**

- **Reconnecting to sensuality through presence**, not performance

- **Embracing inner beauty, wisdom, and the Crone energy in men**—the sage, the guide, the protector

- **Rebuilding psychosexual identity** through integrity, empathy, and spiritual intimacy

Hair loss can catalyze a rebirth—one where **masculinity is no longer performative, but relational**. It challenges outdated paradigms and births new archetypes: the grounded king, the spiritual warrior, the gentle lover.

Therapeutic Tools for Psychosexual Renewal:

- **Narrative Therapy**: Rewriting identity scripts around virility, value, and masculinity

- **Body Image Integration Work**: Mirror practices, somatic self-touch, and movement therapies

- **Psychoeducation**: Teaching the biology of aging and normalizing male hormonal shifts

- **Intimacy Coaching**: Rebuilding relational confidence through authenticity, not appearance

- **Sacred Masculine Rituals**: Ceremonies or mentorship circles for men entering the next phase of life

Hair is not just hair. It's memory, emotion, biology, and story. But it is not identity. In a world obsessed with youthful image, reclaiming inner authority becomes radical. A man who embraces himself—beyond his scalp, skin, or performance—is dangerous in the most beautiful way. He cannot be shamed into silence. He cannot be sold false power.

He *knows* who he is.

Integrative Solutions and Empowered Reframing

Male Pattern Hair Loss (MPHL) may manifest on the surface, but its origins—and its impact—run far deeper. To address it holistically, we must move beyond symptom suppression and into a full-spectrum model of healing: **one that honors the biological terrain, supports emotional resilience, and reclaims self-worth from the inside out**.

> "Hair loss may begin at the follicle, but it ends in the psyche. When we approach it consciously, it becomes a rite of passage—not a source of shame."
> — Dr. Deilen Michelle Villegas

Biological & Functional Strategies: Root Cause Restoration

Rather than defaulting to suppressive pharmaceuticals (like finasteride), functional medicine explores the internal imbalances contributing to MPHL:

1. Functional Lab Testing:

- **Androgen Metabolism Panels:** To assess DHT, testosterone, SHBG, and 5-alpha reductase activity.

- **Micronutrient Analysis:** Checking for deficiencies in zinc, biotin, vitamin D, selenium, and iron (especially ferritin).

- **Inflammation and Thyroid Markers:** Chronic inflammation and subclinical hypothyroidism are often silent contributors to hair loss.

2. Targeted Supplementation:

- **Zinc & Vitamin D:** Vital for testosterone regulation, immune health, and follicle function.

- **Saw Palmetto:** Naturally inhibits 5-alpha-reductase, reducing DHT conversion without suppressing libido like pharmaceuticals.

- **Adaptogens (Ashwagandha, Rhodiola, Reishi):** Lower cortisol, support thyroid health, and reduce stress-driven shedding.

- **Collagen, MSM, and Silica:** Support keratin production and scalp integrity.

3. Scalp & Circulatory Support:

- **Microneedling (Dermarolling):** Stimulates blood flow, collagen, and follicular regeneration.

- **Castor Oil Massage:** Rich in ricinoleic acid and omega-9 fatty acids—promotes circulation and detoxifies scalp tissues.

- **Red Light Therapy:** Emerging evidence shows low-level laser therapy (LLLT) can increase hair density and scalp blood flow.

Rewriting the Mindset: From Hairline to Heartline

Hair loss becomes most damaging not in the body—but in the belief systems men carry about what it means to be *desirable*, *worthy*, or *man enough*. In healing MPHL, mindset work is as critical as any supplement or serum.

Key Reframes for Emotional Empowerment:

- "I am not what is lost—I am what remains."

- "My power is not in how I am seen, but in how I see myself."

- "This shift is not punishment—it's evolution."

Psychosomatic Practices:

- **Mirror Work:** Rebuilding self-image through affirmations and eye contact.

- **Somatic Anchoring:** Connecting to the felt sense of confidence in the body—posture, voice, breath—not just external appearance.

- **Therapeutic Journaling:** Exploring the deeper fears beneath the surface (e.g., "What does hair loss say about me?" and "Is that story true or cultural conditioning?")

Hair Loss as Initiation: A Rite of Passage into Embodied Manhood

What if hair loss was not a decline, but a doorway?

A passage from ego to essence. From external power to

internal presence. From performance-based masculinity to embodied, relational manhood.

Across ancient cultures, physical changes were seen as spiritual invitations. The shedding of hair can symbolize the **stripping of illusions**—the ones that said you had to look a certain way to be valued, loved, or seen.

This chapter in a man's life can become a **reclamation of truth**:

- The truth that **your wisdom is attractive**.

- That **your presence is magnetic**.

- That **your identity is not located on your scalp—it's alive in your soul**.

Integration = Transformation

True healing lies in the integration of science and soul, lab data and legacy, function and feeling. When we treat the root causes and embrace the symbolic shedding, hair loss becomes less of a curse—and more of a calling.

A calling to deeper confidence, awakened masculinity, and an identity rooted not in follicles, but in **fire**.

References

- Ellis, J.A., et al. (2001). The androgen receptor CAG repeat polymorphism and male pattern baldness. *Journal of Investigative Dermatology*, 116(3), 452–455.
- Norwood, O.T. (1975). Male pattern baldness: classification and incidence. *Southern Medical Journal*, 68(11), 1359–1365.
- Randall, V.A. (2008). The endocrine control of the hair follicle. *International Journal of Dermatology*, 47(S2), 20–22.

CHAPTER 11

The Crisis of Traditional Masculinity

Masculinity is not disappearing—it is **evolving**. But that evolution is messy, uncharted, and long overdue.

For generations, men have been handed a script: be strong, be silent, be stoic. Crying was weakness. Vulnerability was shame. Tenderness was emasculation. Especially for Black, Indigenous, and men of color—who often shoulder **historical trauma, hypermasculine expectations, and racialized pressure to appear unbreakable**—the space to be emotionally human has rarely existed.

Now, as cultural norms shift and the collective nervous system of our society begins to unravel the old stories, **modern men are left standing between two worlds**: the old model of power through suppression and the emerging path of power through self-awareness, emotional literacy, and relational presence.

> "The old story said 'don't feel.' The new story says 'feel—and rise.'" — Dr. Deilen Michelle Villegas

The Crisis Beneath the Surface

While public discourse focuses on gender roles, identity politics, and toxic masculinity, the **quiet crisis** facing men is rarely addressed at the root.

Emotional Suppression as Survival

From a young age, boys are socialized to suppress their emotions. Phrases like "man up," "don't be soft," or "stop acting like a girl" teach them that feeling is dangerous. Over time, the suppression of grief, fear, sadness, and tenderness becomes not just cultural—but **neurological**. Emotional numbing turns into nervous system dysregulation, poor relational communication, and chronic health issues.

Performative Strength and Identity Exhaustion

Strength is often measured by how much a man can endure, not how deeply he can feel. This leads to performance-based self-worth: productivity over presence, sex over intimacy, domination over connection. Many men feel they must *achieve* manhood daily—never allowed to simply be.

Social Media, Comparison, and Censorship

In the digital age, social media has both exposed and distorted masculinity. Men compare themselves to filtered physiques, exaggerated lifestyles, or hyper-aggressive male influencers promoting emotional detachment as power. And when men *do* open up online, they are often met with ridicule, censorship, or invalidation—especially if their vulnerability challenges traditional gender norms or cultural expectations.

⚠ BIPOC Men and the "Strong Black/Brown Male" Mythology

For BIPOC men, the weight is even heavier. Centuries of systemic racism, over-policing, and generational trauma have forced them into hardened archetypes of resilience. The world expects them to be bulletproof—but then punishes them for being too "aggressive," "stoic," or "broken." In reality, these men are often navigating **unacknowledged grief, inherited fear, and survival-based masculinity** without tools, space, or language to name it.

The Neurobiology of Male Emotional Pain

The male brain is often wired for action—but not trained for reflection. Prolonged emotional suppression can lead to:

- **HPA axis dysregulation** (chronic stress and cortisol elevation)

- **Reduced oxytocin and emotional bonding**

- **Heightened inflammation and depression masked as irritability, addiction, or withdrawal**

And when men are discouraged from seeking help, these symptoms worsen in silence.

The New Masculine Paradigm: Power With, Not Power Over

Masculinity is not toxic—**suppression is.**

We are not asking men to become less masculine. We are inviting them to become **fully human**—to reclaim the parts of themselves long buried under shame, fear, and societal pressure.

The new masculine archetype is:

- Emotionally attuned

- Spiritually connected

- Relationally responsible

- Grounded in presence, not performance

This redefinition honors *both the warrior and the healer, the protector and the nurturer, the assertive and the vulnerable.*

Healing Masculinity in BIPOC Communities

Restoring modern manhood—especially for men of color—requires:

- **Culturally relevant mental health spaces**

- **Trauma-informed, somatic-based healing frameworks**

- **Mentorship and storytelling circles led by emotionally**

evolved men

- **Reconnection with ancestral masculine wisdom that honors feeling, ritual, and balance**

  "Our ancestors did not raise boys into men through suppression—they guided them through **rites of passage**, emotional preparation, and sacred responsibility."

Masculinity is Not Ending. It's Awakening.

This chapter isn't about what men have lost—it's about what they are on the verge of reclaiming:

- **Permission to feel**

- **The right to heal**

- **The courage to be whole**

This is the second initiation. Not into domination—but into **integration.**

Masculinity is not found in the armor—it's found in the courage to take it off.

Emotional Suppression, Gender Role Conditioning, and Internalized Shame in Men: A Psychosocial and Neurobiological Review

Traditional gender socialization processes have long reinforced the suppression of emotional expression in boys and men. From early developmental stages, males are often conditioned through explicit and implicit messaging to "man up," avoid crying, and equate strength with emotional stoicism. This phenomenon is culturally reinforced across media, peer groups, and familial systems, forming what Mahalik et al. (2003) term *restrictive emotionality*—a key component of traditional masculine ideology.

While intended to promote resilience, these prescriptions often result in psychological fragmentation, not integration. Emotional suppression, particularly of grief, fear, and vulnerability, does not result in the extinguishment of those emotional states. Rather, it leads to their displacement into maladaptive coping strategies such as compulsive achievement, substance misuse, aggression, emotional withdrawal, or somatic symptoms (Levant et al., 2009; Addis & Mahalik, 2003). Suppressed affect has also been linked to increased allostatic load, hypothalamic-pituitary-adrenal (HPA) axis dysregulation, and inflammatory cytokine elevation, which contribute to mood disorders, cardiovascular risk, and immune dysfunction (Sapolsky, 2004; Slavich & Irwin, 2014).

Rigid gender role schemas—particularly the triad of the *stoic provider*, *protector*, and *problem-solver*—leave little room for emotional nuance or relational interdependence. This model falsely assumes that vulnerability equates to weakness and that self-worth must be externally validated through performance and dominance. Consequently, many men internalize shame when their lived emotional experience deviates from these expectations, reinforcing disconnection from the self and others. Brown (2007) identifies shame as the core affective consequence of failing to meet gender-based social expectations, often leading to concealment, isolation, and a diminished capacity for intimacy.

In clinical contexts, this dissonance between authentic self and performed identity frequently presents as masked depression, emotional dysregulation, or relational dissatisfaction. Men may describe burnout, numbness, or persistent irritability, yet score below diagnostic thresholds for major depression due to the externalized and somatized presentation of their symptoms (Martin et al., 2013).

Relationship conflicts may be driven by an inability to articulate emotional needs or respond empathically to those of others, reflecting underdeveloped affective language and somatic attunement.

Moreover, performance-based self-worth—wherein a man's value is defined by output, productivity, or control—limits emotional resilience and reinforces achievement-based validation patterns. This mode of existence, while societally rewarded, is psychospiritually unsustainable, often culminating in midlife crises, somatic collapse, or emotional estrangement.

Implications for Practice

Therapeutic interventions must attend to the culturally embedded scripts of masculinity and their neurological and relational consequences. Somatic therapies, narrative reprocessing, and group-based emotional literacy programs can aid in deconstructing internalized shame while facilitating embodied self-awareness and interpersonal attunement. Creating gender-affirming spaces that decouple masculinity from emotional suppression is essential in promoting holistic well-being among male-identifying clients.

Social Media, Masculinity, and the Crisis of Curated Identity

In the digital age, platforms such as Instagram, TikTok, YouTube, and X (formerly Twitter) have emerged as powerful forces shaping modern identity formation—particularly for men navigating questions of self-worth, status, and masculinity. While these platforms offer opportunities for connection and creativity, they also perpetuate distorted and often harmful ideals of what it means to "be a man." The result is a growing dissonance between authentic selfhood and digitally mediated expectation.

Social media rewards performative masculinity: the curated display of wealth, physical dominance, sexual prowess, and unemotional control. These metrics—likes, shares, virality —become external validators of internal worth. For many men, especially adolescents and young adults, these digital environments set unrealistic and narrow standards of success. The algorithm favors aesthetics over authenticity, spectacle over substance. Vulnerability is often penalized, while hypermasculine tropes are amplified.

This curated masculinity reinforces a dangerous paradigm: that a man's value is proportional to his body, his bank account, or his ability to perform sexually and socially. What remains hidden beneath these images is the emotional cost— burnout, disconnection, dysmorphia, and deep-rooted shame.

Research highlights the psychological toll. A 2014 study by Pantic found a direct correlation between time spent on social media and increased symptoms of depression and lowered self-esteem in male users, particularly when platforms were used for social comparison. More recent studies have emphasized that young men who consume content centered around "alpha male" culture, aesthetic fitness, or wealth accumulation report higher levels of anxiety, dissatisfaction, and social withdrawal (Fardouly et al., 2015; Griffiths et al., 2018).

Additionally, the male body image crisis is rising. While female-centered body dysmorphia has been extensively studied, emerging research shows that exposure to idealized male physiques online contributes to muscle dysmorphia, disordered eating, steroid use, and compulsive exercise in men (Murray et al., 2017). The gap between one's real body and the sculpted, filtered bodies seen online becomes a source of silent shame—one that is rarely acknowledged in mainstream discourse.

Perhaps most concerning is that for many young men, social media has become a *primary* education on what manhood is supposed to look like—bypassing community elders, spiritual frameworks, or lived emotional experiences. This bypass can create a generation of men who are externally polished but internally fragmented.

Clinical and Educational Implications

- **Therapeutic Inquiry**: Clinicians should assess social media habits during intake, exploring how these platforms influence a client's body image, relationship expectations, and self-esteem.

- **Digital Detox and Media Literacy**: Encouraging periods of intentional disconnection and critical analysis of social media content can help clients reclaim narrative agency and reduce toxic comparison.

- **Reframing Masculine Identity**: Facilitating group dialogues or workshops that challenge algorithmic masculinity and promote relational, spiritual, and creative dimensions of manhood can serve as powerful tools for healing.

Censorship, Isolation, and Sexuality: The Silencing of Male Intimacy

The discourse around male sexuality remains profoundly constrained by cultural taboos, gender stereotypes, and social policing. While society has made strides in destigmatizing female sexual empowerment and mental health, discussions about men's emotional, sensual, and psychosexual well-being are still met with discomfort, ridicule, or outright censorship —especially when they diverge from heteronormative, performance-driven models of masculinity.

The Policing of Pleasure

From early childhood, boys are conditioned to pursue pleasure through domination rather than connection. Touch, when not explicitly sexualized, is often discouraged. Emotional intimacy between men is rare and, in many cases, pathologized. Expressions of tenderness, curiosity, or embodied sensuality—such as emotional touch, conscious breathing, or prostate stimulation—are labeled as "feminine," "weak," or "deviant." This fear of feminization is a direct byproduct of patriarchal structures that equate vulnerability with inferiority.

Sexual exploration that deviates from the mainstream is not only socially punished but algorithmically censored. On social media platforms and digital forums, content that promotes energy-based sexuality (such as tantra), queer-inclusive pleasure practices, or somatic intimacy is often shadowbanned or removed. This digital censorship reinforces a narrow vision of male sexuality—one centered on penetration, performance, and control—leaving no room for emotional depth, spiritual connection, or alternative pathways to arousal.

The Isolation Epidemic

The consequences of this censorship extend beyond the sexual domain. Emotional isolation among men is reaching epidemic levels. Studies consistently show that men report fewer close friendships, engage in less emotional disclosure, and are less likely to seek mental health support compared to women (Mahalik et al., 2003). The COVID-19 pandemic exacerbated this trend, further cutting men off from communal spaces, physical touch, and rites of passage that once anchored masculine identity.

This systemic disconnection is not without consequence.

Globally, men are more likely to die by suicide, with middle-aged men being particularly vulnerable (WHO, 2021). These statistics point not only to untreated depression but to a deeper cultural grief: a profound loss of emotional literacy, meaningful connection, and sacred sexuality.

The Need for Psychosexual Liberation

If we are to support the whole man, we must create environments where diverse expressions of male intimacy are not only allowed but encouraged. This includes:

- **Normalizing Non-Linear Pleasure**: Teaching men that sexuality is not about performance but about presence and sensation.

- **Validating Emotional Sensuality**: Creating language and rituals that allow men to feel safe in their bodies and desires.

- **Expanding Clinical Conversations**: Inviting men to explore psychosexual healing as part of trauma recovery, hormone optimization, and nervous system regulation.

In somatic sex therapy and trauma-informed care, male clients often report a sense of "returning home" when they experience touch without agenda, when their bodies are allowed to soften, and when pleasure is decoupled from performance. For many, this is the first time they have been given permission to be both sensual and safe.

Clinical Reflection: Supporting Male Clients in Reclaiming Sexual Sovereignty

- **Ask deeper questions**: How do you feel about your body when you're not performing? What were you taught about touch, intimacy, or pleasure as a child?

- **Use inclusive language**: Offer alternatives to "dominance" and "control" as masculine ideals. Introduce concepts like attunement, presence, and vulnerability as strengths.

- **Normalize exploration**: Encourage experimentation with non-traditional pleasure modalities in a nonjudgmental, trauma-informed context.

Reclaiming male sexuality from censorship, isolation, and performative scripts is not just an act of healing—it's an act of liberation. When men are free to feel, explore, and express without shame, they not only heal themselves—they disrupt generational patterns and create space for deeper, more conscious relationships. As practitioners, clinicians, and cultural architects, our role is not to prescribe what masculinity should be—but to hold space for what it *can* become.

Toward a New Masculine Archetype: Wholeness as Strength

The cultural crisis of masculinity is not a call for men to abandon their power—it's an invitation to *reclaim* it in its wholeness. For too long, masculinity has been narrowly defined through domination, stoicism, and performance, severing men from their inner worlds and spiritual depth. But a new masculine archetype is rising—one rooted not in suppression or superiority, but in embodiment, emotional integrity, and soulful leadership.

This new masculine is not fragile. He is forged in the fire of truth-telling and tempered by the courage to feel. He does not need to dominate to feel powerful—his presence is his power. He does not fear vulnerability—he knows it is the birthplace of connection, authenticity, and sacred intimacy.

Integration Over Imitation

Healing the masculine does not mean abandoning masculine traits—it means *integrating* them. It means holding discipline in one hand and emotional literacy in the other. It means wielding the sword of discernment without severing from compassion. The new masculine archetype includes the Warrior, yes—but also the Mystic, the Steward, the Father, the Lover, and the Elder.

This integration invites men to reclaim all parts of themselves:

- The fierce protector *and* the gentle nurturer

- The provider *and* the present partner

- The logical thinker *and* the intuitive feeler

- The sensual body *and* the spiritual being

This is not about emasculation—it's about expansion.

A New Framework for the Evolved Man

To move toward this integrated model, men are called to:

Seek Mentorship and Emotional Support

Healing is not solitary. Whether through brotherhood circles, therapy, ancestral traditions, or rites of passage, men must reclaim the power of interdependence. Vulnerability among men builds trust, safety, and community—the antidotes to isolation and shame.

Explore Non-Traditional Healing Practices

Breathwork, somatic therapy, plant medicine, tantra, meditation, and energy work offer men tools to regulate their nervous systems and reconnect with their bodies—especially after years of numbing or performance-based conditioning.

Release Shame Around Sexuality, Appearance, and Failure

The new masculine recognizes that self-worth is not rooted in hairlines, bank accounts, or sexual conquests. It is rooted in embodiment, relational depth, and self-awareness. Shame dissolves when men are seen and celebrated in their full humanity—not just their utility.

Reparent the Inner Boy and Heal Ancestral Wounds

Many men carry the emotional bruises of absent fathers, emotionally unavailable mothers, or inherited trauma from generations who could not safely express emotion. Reconnecting with the inner child allows men to heal the parts that still seek validation, safety, and love.

Redefine Power Through Presence

Rather than power over, the new masculine models *power with* —in relationships, communities, and within the self. He does not hustle to earn worth. He *knows* his worth and brings that grounded knowing into every room, every decision, and every touch.

The Sacred Masculine in Practice

This shift is already happening—in boardrooms where conscious leaders are integrating emotional intelligence, in therapy rooms where men cry for the first time in decades, in bedrooms where intimacy is finally rooted in safety rather than conquest, and in healing circles where men gather not to perform but to be *seen*.

As we dismantle the outdated scripts, we make room for a masculinity that is *authentic, anchored*, and *alive*. A masculinity that heals, not harms. That creates, not conquers. That speaks truth, holds space, and protects the sacred.

The new masculine is not a destination—it is a becoming.

It is the man who is unafraid to feel.

It is the father who listens before he teaches.

It is the leader who regulates his nervous system before he raises his voice.

It is the partner who meets you with presence, not projection.

It is the man who is no longer confined by who he was taught to be—

but who dares to remember who he truly is.

References

- Pantic, I. (2014). Online social networking and mental health. *Cyberpsychology, Behavior, and Social Networking*, 17(10), 652–657.
- Mahalik, J.R., et al. (2003). Masculinity and perceived normative health behaviors. *Journal of Men's Health & Gender*, 1(2), 139–144.
- Wong, Y.J., et al. (2017). Meta-analyses of the relationship between conformity to masculine norms and mental health-related outcomes. *Journal of Counseling Psychology*, 64(1), 80–93.
- World Health Organization (WHO). (2021). *Suicide worldwide in 2019: Global health estimates.*
- Diamond, L. M., & Huebner, D. M. (2012). Is good sex good for you? Rethinking sexuality and health. *Social and Personality Psychology Compass*, 6(1), 54–69.
- Fardouly, J., Diedrichs, P. C., Vartanian, L. R., & Halliwell, E. (2015). Social comparisons on social media: The impact of Facebook on young women's body image concerns and mood. *Body Image*, 13, 38–45.
- Griffiths, S., Murray, S. B., Krug, I., & McLean, S. A. (2018). The contribution of social media to body dissatisfaction, eating disorder symptoms, and anabolic steroid use

among sexual minority men. *Cyberpsychology, Behavior, and Social Networking, 21*(3), 149–156.

- Murray, S. B., Rieger, E., Hildebrandt, T., Karlov, L., & Russell, J. (2017). A comparison of eating, exercise, shape, and weight-related symptoms in males with muscle dysmorphia and anorexia nervosa. *Body Image, 10*(3), 290–293.

- Addis, M. E., & Mahalik, J. R. (2003). Men, masculinity, and the contexts of help seeking. *American Psychologist, 58*(1), 5–14.

- Brown, B. (2007). *I Thought It Was Just Me (But It Isn't): Telling the Truth About Perfectionism, Inadequacy, and Power.* Penguin.

- Levant, R. F., Hall, R. J., & Rankin, T. J. (2009). Male role norms inventory-short form (MRNI-SF): Development, confirmatory factor analytic investigation of structure, and measurement invariance. *Journal of Counseling Psychology, 56*(4), 573–587.

- Martin, L. A., Neighbors, H. W., & Griffith, D. M. (2013). The experience of symptoms of depression in men vs. women: Analysis of the National Comorbidity Survey Replication. *JAMA Psychiatry, 70*(10), 1100–1106.

- Sapolsky, R. M. (2004). *Why Zebras Don't Get Ulcers.* Holt Paperbacks.

- Slavich, G. M., & Irwin, M. R. (2014). From stress to inflammation and major depressive disorder: A social signal transduction theory of depression. *Psychological Bulletin, 140*(3), 774–815.

CHAPTER 12

Prostate Health, Erectile
Function & True Libido

Beyond Performance, Into Presence

Sexual health in men is often reduced to performance, stamina, and penetration. But beneath the cultural obsession with erections lies a deeper need for intimacy, vitality, and self-connection. Here we will explore the anatomy and energetic function of the prostate, the rise of erectile dysfunction (ED), and how to reframe libido as more than just physical desire. By restoring sexual wellness through a holistic lens, we can invite men back into embodied masculinity rooted in presence—not pressure.

> "True libido is not just the hunger for sex—it's the body's call to feel, to connect, to be alive." — Dr. Deilen Michelle Villegas

The Prostate: Anatomical and Energetic Overview

The prostate may be small in size, but its influence on male health, vitality, and identity is monumental. Nestled just below the bladder and encircling the urethra, this walnut-sized gland plays a key role in reproductive function—producing seminal fluid that nourishes and transports sperm during ejaculation. Yet its relevance extends far beyond physiology.

Energetically, the prostate is a root center of masculine power—closely tied to grounding, sexuality, creative life force, and unprocessed emotion. In somatic and ancestral traditions, this area of the male body is where rage, grief, fear, and suppressed desire often reside. When tension accumulates here, it can manifest not only as physical dysfunction but as emotional disconnection, shame, or sexual shutdown.

Common Prostate Concerns: Beyond the Physical

Prostate issues are increasingly common, especially as men age—but they are rarely explored in a holistic or trauma-informed way. Understanding the intersection between biology and biography is essential to unraveling the full story.

Benign Prostatic Hyperplasia (BPH)

An enlarged prostate that restricts urinary flow, leading to nocturia (nighttime urination), hesitancy, and incomplete emptying. While often attributed to aging, BPH is also influenced by inflammation, hormonal imbalance (especially DHT), and poor lymphatic circulation.

Prostatitis

Inflammation of the prostate, which may be bacterial or non-bacterial. In holistic medicine, non-bacterial prostatitis is often associated with stress, unresolved trauma, or sexual frustration. Clients with a history of sexual shame, chronic pelvic tension, or emotional repression often present with these symptoms.

Prostate Cancer

The second most common cancer among men globally. While genetics play a role, environmental toxins, dietary habits, chronic inflammation, and emotional stagnation in the pelvic floor are also major contributors.

Risk Factors: A Multifactorial Reality

Prostate dysfunction doesn't arise in a vacuum. It reflects years of layered stressors—some physical, others emotional or spiritual.

- **Age over 50:** Hormonal changes, cumulative exposure to

toxins, and inflammation increase over time.

- **Family history**: Genetic predisposition may influence risk, but epigenetic expression is largely shaped by environment and lifestyle.

- **Dietary patterns**: High consumption of animal fats, alcohol, and processed foods increases inflammation and oxidative stress.

- **Environmental toxins**: Exposure to endocrine-disrupting chemicals (plastics, pesticides, heavy metals) affects testosterone and DHT metabolism.

- **Emotional stagnation**: Unexpressed anger, grief, or shame can become energetically "stored" in the pelvic region, contributing to dysfunction.

- **Pelvic trauma**: Injury, surgery, or sexual trauma can disrupt nerve signaling, tissue function, and energetic flow in the region.

Energetics of the Prostate: The Masculine Root

In many Indigenous and Eastern systems, the pelvic basin is considered the seat of life force energy, or *chi/prana*. The prostate, in particular, aligns with the **root and sacral chakras**, governing themes such as:

- Grounding and physical security

- Sexuality and reproductive power

- Emotional resilience and containment

- Creativity and sacred masculinity

When a man feels ungrounded, emasculated, disconnected from pleasure, or burdened by shame, the prostate often mirrors these imbalances. This is why emotional and energetic care must be part of every integrative approach to prostate health.

Supportive Practices for Prostate Wellness

Restoring prostate vitality involves more than symptom management—it requires a full-body recalibration. The following practices help address the biological, lifestyle, and emotional roots of prostate concerns.

Nutrition & Anti-Inflammatory Support

- Emphasize **cruciferous vegetables** (broccoli, cauliflower, kale) to support estrogen metabolism and detoxification.

- Include **omega-3 fatty acids, green tea**, and **turmeric** to reduce inflammation.

- Reduce or eliminate **dairy, alcohol, red meat**, and refined sugar, which can worsen inflammation and hormone imbalance.

Targeted Supplementation

- **Zinc**: Crucial for testosterone metabolism and prostate tissue integrity.

- **Selenium**: Supports antioxidant activity and cancer prevention.

- **Saw Palmetto**: Traditionally used to reduce DHT activity and improve urinary flow.

- **Quercetin**: Supports inflammation reduction and is

especially helpful for prostatitis.

Physical Movement & Pelvic Activation

- Practice **pelvic floor exercises** (e.g., Kegels for men) to enhance circulation and nerve function.

- Incorporate **castor oil packs**, **rebounding**, or **dry brushing** to support lymphatic flow.

- Regular **ejaculation** promotes prostate fluid turnover and reduces congestion. However, intentional celibacy periods paired with energy practices (like tantra or breathwork) may also serve prostate energetics in specific healing journeys.

Somatic & Energetic Healing

- **Somatic therapy and trauma-informed bodywork** help release stored tension and unprocessed emotional trauma from the pelvic floor.

- **Breathwork and meditation** grounded in the root chakra enhance self-trust and embodied presence.

- **Tantric or Taoist practices** teach men how to circulate sexual energy through the whole body, preventing stagnation in the prostate area.

Reclaiming Masculine Vitality

The prostate is more than an anatomical gland—it is an emotional and spiritual compass. When men begin to honor this part of themselves, not as a problem to be fixed but a portal to deeper self-knowing, healing accelerates. Men are not taught to *listen* to their pelvic floor—but when they do, they often rediscover their power, presence, and purpose.

"A healthy prostate is not just the absence of disease

—it is the presence of integrated masculinity, embodied pleasure, and emotional fluency." — Dr. Deilen MichelleVillegas

The Pleasure Function of the Prostate

Beyond reproduction, the prostate is also a powerful center of sexual pleasure. Sometimes referred to as the "male G-spot," the prostate can generate euphoric sensations when stimulated—often described as deeper, fuller, and more encompassing than penile orgasms alone. This pleasure is a direct result of its rich network of nerve endings and its role in the body's natural sexual response.

Many heterosexual men report enjoying prostate stimulation, whether through partnered play or solo exploration. However, because of the prostate's anatomical location—accessible through the anus—there is significant social stigma attached to this form of pleasure. Cultural homophobia, rigid gender norms, and misinformation have led to the shaming of men who explore their bodies in this way.

> "Enjoying prostate stimulation does not indicate sexual orientation—it honors the human body's capacity for pleasure." – Dr. Deilen Michelle Viilegas

Prostate pleasure is about anatomy, not identity. Its enjoyment is not inherently linked to being gay or straight, but rather to a man's relationship with his own body and his openness to deeper sensation. Dismantling this stigma allows men to reclaim full-spectrum pleasure and release shame about their natural design.

Educating clients about the anatomy and function of the prostate is essential for sexual healing and empowerment. When discussed openly and with respect, prostate exploration can become a path to profound intimacy, emotional release, and even spiritual awakening.

Erectile Dysfunction: A Symptom, Not an Identity

Erectile dysfunction (ED) is one of the most emotionally charged and misunderstood symptoms men face—yet it is incredibly common. An estimated **30 million men** in the U.S. experience ED, and rates are rising among those **under 40**, especially in BIPOC and trauma-affected communities. Despite its prevalence, ED continues to carry immense stigma, often silently eroding confidence, relationships, and mental health.

ED is not a singular diagnosis—it is a *somatic signal*, a reflection of deeper imbalances in the body, mind, and emotional nervous system. Too often, men internalize ED as a sign of failure or weakness, rather than viewing it as a *symptom of dysregulation or disconnection*.

> "Erectile dysfunction is not a loss of manhood—it is a message from the body asking to be heard, held, and healed." — Dr. Deilen Michelle Villegas

Key Contributors to Erectile Dysfunction

Rather than viewing ED solely through the lens of aging or physical disease, it is more accurate—and more healing—to approach it holistically. These are some of the most common and clinically observed contributors:

Poor Blood Flow & Endothelial Dysfunction

Healthy erections rely on optimal blood flow. Conditions like **hypertension, insulin resistance, and high cholesterol** compromise the vascular system, impeding circulation to the penis and reducing erectile function.

Low Testosterone or Elevated SHBG

Declining free testosterone levels, common with stress, aging, and poor lifestyle, reduce libido and erectile strength. Elevated **Sex Hormone-Binding Globulin (SHBG)** further reduces bioavailable testosterone, impacting sensitivity and desire.

Prescription Medications

Medications—especially **SSRIs, beta blockers, statins,** and some antihypertensives—can interfere with sexual function by disrupting neurotransmitter or vascular pathways.

Porn-Induced Desensitization (PIED)

The rise in **porn-induced erectile dysfunction** is a growing concern. Repeated exposure to hyperstimulating, digitally curated content trains the brain to associate arousal with artificial novelty rather than real-world intimacy. This leads to **dopamine burnout, performance anxiety**, and emotional disconnection during partnered sex.

Performance Anxiety & Emotional Trauma

Unresolved **sexual trauma, shame, or relational insecurity** can embed deep in the nervous system, creating unconscious tension and withdrawal. This internalized fear often manifests during intimacy, making the body feel unsafe or unable to fully relax and engage.

Case Study: Jalen's Return to Sensation

Jalen, a 36-year-old Black entrepreneur, sought counseling after months of difficulty maintaining erections. Despite being physically healthy and successful in his career, he felt a growing sense of inadequacy, isolation, and fear of being seen as "broken."

Initial Clinical Findings:

- Normal cardiovascular screening

- Borderline low free testosterone, elevated SHBG

- Daily porn use since adolescence

- History of childhood sexual boundary violation

- High stress, minimal sleep, and chronic tension in the pelvic floor

Jalen's symptoms weren't just physical—they were *neurological, emotional, and relational.*

Healing Plan: A Holistic, Integrative Approach

Jalen's healing journey focused on regulation, reconnection, and reclamation:

Somatic & Pelvic Therapy

- **Breathwork and vagal toning** to shift from sympathetic overdrive to parasympathetic safety

- **Pelvic floor therapy** to release tension, restore circulation, and reawaken nerve pathways

- **Guided body scan meditations** to reestablish internal awareness of pleasure and sensation

Erotic Rewiring

- Abstinence from pornography to allow for **neuroplastic repair of arousal circuits**

- Conscious re-engagement with fantasy through **touch, visualization**, and emotional intimacy

- Exploration of pleasure without the pressure of performance, allowing arousal to reemerge naturally

Emotional Processing & Trauma Integration

- Inner child work and narrative therapy around his early experiences of shame and violation

- Reframing his self-worth beyond sexual function

- Rebuilding trust in his body and in safe relational dynamics

Nutritional & Herbal Support

- **L-arginine and beetroot** to support nitric oxide and vasodilation

- **Panax ginseng and maca root** to enhance energy, libido, and endocrine balance

- Targeted nutrients: **zinc, vitamin D3, and magnesium**

Breakthrough and New Beginnings

By month three, Jalen began experiencing **spontaneous erections** and reported a dramatic shift in emotional confidence. He entered a new relationship rooted in **emotional connection, honesty, and mutual safety**—one where sex was no longer a performance, but a shared experience of presence and pleasure.

> "I stopped chasing the erection and started listening to my body. I didn't just get my sex life back—I found parts of myself I didn't even know were missing." — Jalen

ED Is a Portal, Not a Punishment

What if ED wasn't something to fear—but something to *honor*?

When men learn to decode the language of the body, ED becomes an opportunity to:

- Heal the nervous system

- Explore emotional intimacy

- Reclaim self-worth beyond sexual performance

- Align sexuality with truth, not pressure

The journey of healing erectile dysfunction is not just about achieving erections—it's about restoring *embodiment, empowerment, and connection.*

Libido: A Multifactorial Reflection of Health and Wholeness

Libido is often narrowly defined through the lens of testosterone—but male sexual desire is far more complex than a single hormone. Libido is an *energetic barometer*, influenced not only by biology but by a man's emotional landscape, relational dynamics, and overall sense of vitality and purpose.

Sexual desire does not exist in a vacuum. It is responsive, relational, and deeply sensitive to both internal neurochemistry and external stressors.

> "A man's libido is not just about performance—it is a reflection of how alive, aligned, and emotionally resourced he feels." — Dr. Deilen Michelle Villegas

Beyond Testosterone: The Full Spectrum of Libido Drivers

While testosterone plays an important role in initiating sexual desire and erectile response, it is only *one* piece of a much larger physiological and emotional puzzle. Other key hormones and neurotransmitters include:

Dopamine

Often called the "motivation molecule," dopamine fuels *desire, pursuit, and novelty*. Low dopamine—common in men with chronic stress, pornography overuse, or depression—can dull interest in sex and reduce overall pleasure response.

Oxytocin

The "bonding hormone" released during touch, orgasm, and emotional connection. When oxytocin is low, sex may feel mechanical or emotionally distant, even in long-term relationships.

Cortisol

Chronically high cortisol levels (due to stress, trauma, or overwork) **suppress testosterone** and create a state of *sympathetic dominance*—where the body is in fight-or-flight, not rest-and-receive. This physiological state is inherently anti-pleasure.

Thyroid Hormones

Hypothyroidism can result in fatigue, depression, and low libido. T3 and T4 also regulate metabolic rate and mood—both of which are key to maintaining healthy sexual desire and stamina.

Psychological and Emotional State

Libido is deeply affected by **grief, relational disconnection, trauma, shame, and loss of purpose**. Men navigating identity shifts, burnout, or emotional suppression may experience a libido drop not due to dysfunction, but disembodiment.

Rebuilding Libido Holistically

Rather than chasing testosterone levels alone, a holistic approach to restoring libido honors the *mind-body-spirit connection* of male vitality.

Increase Dopamine Naturally

- Engage in **purpose-driven activities** that bring meaning

- Get **daily sunlight and movement**

- Cultivate **novelty and play**: new music, books,

adventures

- Celebrate small wins to rewire reward pathways

Reduce Cortisol and Reconnect to Safety

- **Breathwork** (box breathing, 4-7-8 method) to calm the nervous system

- Time in **nature** to reset circadian and hormonal rhythms

- Honor **boundaries** with work, tech, and toxic relationships

- Prioritize **restorative sleep** and screen-free evenings

Herbal and Nutritional Allies

- **Maca root**: Increases energy, libido, and sperm count

- **Tongkat Ali**: Enhances free testosterone and mood

- **Tribulus Terrestris**: Supports luteinizing hormone and libido

- **Horny Goat Weed (Epimedium)**: Increases nitric oxide and circulation

Note: All herbs should be used under the guidance of a practitioner, especially for those with pre-existing conditions or medications.

Explore Sensuality Beyond Sexuality

Often, the fastest way to reclaim libido is not through performance—but through **presence**. Men who feel numb, shut down, or emotionally disconnected may benefit from practices that restore **embodied pleasure**, including:

- **Sensual massage** (solo or partnered)

- **Ecstatic dance** or conscious movement

- **Art, music, or cooking** as creative expressions of life force

- **Eye-gazing, breathwork, or tantra** to reestablish intimacy and self-trust

Case Insight: Rekindling Desire After Burnout

One client, a 41-year-old educator navigating career stress and fatherhood, reported feeling "asexual" and guilty about his lack of interest in intimacy. Lab results were normal, but emotionally he felt **disconnected from himself and uninspired in his relationship**.

We focused on:

- **Dopamine-rich habits**: morning walks, spontaneous date nights, creating music

- **Sensate focus exercises** with his partner—non-sexual touch and mindfulness

- **Adaptogenic support** (rhodiola, ashwagandha) to regulate cortisol

- **Somatic journaling** around unspoken resentments and grief

In 6 weeks, he reported feeling "like myself again," and intimacy naturally returned—without force or performance pressure.

The Takeaway: Libido is Aliveness

When a man feels safe in his body, connected to his emotions, and purposeful in his life—libido often returns. It is not something to chase or fear losing. It is something to *tend*, like a sacred fire.

Visual: Root Causes of Erectile Dysfunction and Holistic Interventions

Root Cause	Physical or Emotional Symptom	Supportive Therapy
Vascular/Metabolic	Poor circulation, weak erections	Cardio, nitric oxide boosters
Hormonal	Low libido, fatigue, mood swings	Hormone testing, herbs, strength training
Nervous System Trauma	Performance anxiety, numbness	Somatic therapy, EMDR, pelvic bodywork
Psychological/Relational	Disconnection, shame, trust issues	Couples therapy, self-esteem work

The Sacred Masculine and Sexual Embodiment

Sexual energy is not separate from spiritual energy—it *is* spiritual energy, expressed through the body. It is life force. Creative fire. The same current that sparks conception also fuels innovation, leadership, connection, and presence. In the body of the Sacred Masculine, this energy becomes not just a vehicle for pleasure or procreation, but a portal for profound embodiment and transformation.

> "The most erotic part of a man is his presence." — Dr. Deilen Michelle Villegas

Reclaiming the Erotic as Sacred

In a society obsessed with performance and aesthetics, many men have internalized a disconnected model of sexuality—one where pleasure is goal-oriented, disconnected from emotion, and stripped of reverence. But sacred sexuality invites a return to the body as *temple*, not machine.

When men dissociate from their bodies due to trauma, shame, or overexposure to performance-based intimacy (pornography, hypermasculine ideals), their sexual energy becomes either compulsive or absent. Desire is no longer a whisper from the soul—it becomes a burden, a race, or a void.

True sexual embodiment begins when a man turns inward and reclaims his eroticism as an expression of aliveness, not proof of masculinity.

The Role of Presence in Erotic Power

Presence is the most magnetic, arousing, and healing quality a man can bring into intimacy. It is the ability to **be fully in the moment**—to feel, to witness, to respond, not just with the body, but with the heart and nervous system attuned.

Presence says:

- *"I am here."*

- *"I am safe."*

- *"I see you."*

- *"I feel myself."*

This presence creates safety—not just for a partner, but for the man himself. In this space, vulnerability becomes powerful, and intimacy becomes a ritual of mutual unfolding.

Erotic Energy as Healing Energy

Sexual energy, when unblocked, is not chaotic—it is intelligent. It holds the potential to:

- **Heal trauma** through embodied pleasure

- **Restore nervous system balance** by releasing endorphins and oxytocin

- **Deepen spiritual practice**, especially when guided through tantric breathwork or conscious touch

- **Rebuild self-worth**, reminding men they are not just performers—they are *receivers* of love and pleasure, too

In somatic therapy, many male clients report feeling "numb from the waist down" or "cut off from their desire." This is not dysfunction—it is *protection*. And with the right guidance, this numbness can soften into sensitivity, sensation, and self-intimacy.

Practices of Sacred Embodiment

To awaken the Sacred Masculine, men must learn to *feel* again. Not just physically—but emotionally, sensually, spiritually.

Practices to Cultivate Sacred Embodiment:

- **Tantric breathwork** to circulate life force and expand pleasure

- **Somatic awareness** of the pelvic floor, hips, and heart center

- **Sensate focus exercises** to rewire the brain-body connection

- **Self-touch with presence**, free of goal or climax

- **Ritual intimacy** that includes eye-gazing, intention setting, and slowing down

- **Emotional integration**: journaling, crying, sounding, moving through grief and shame

Protecting vs. Penetrating: A Rebalanced Masculine

In the archetype of the Sacred Masculine, sexual energy is not about conquest—it is about **connection**. It is not about taking —it is about *being received with integrity*. This is the erotic maturity our world desperately needs.

When men begin to embody their sexual energy with consciousness:

- They become better lovers

- More present fathers

- More intuitive leaders

- And more authentic versions of themselves

Sacred Union Begins Within

Ultimately, sexual embodiment is not just for relational connection—it is for **self-union**. When a man can meet his own desire without shame, hold his own arousal with reverence, and honor his own body as divine, *he becomes whole*.

And from that wholeness, all else flows—pleasure, passion, purpose, partnership.

The Pulse of Pleasure, the Path to Power

Healing sexual function is not simply about fixing what's "broken." It's about reclaiming something far more profound —**a man's relationship with his own life force**. Sexual health is a mirror. It reflects not just physical status, but emotional well-being, nervous system regulation, self-image, relational dynamics, and spiritual vitality.

Prostate health, erectile integrity, and libido are not isolated issues—they are *vital signs* of how well a man is tending to the temple of his body, the state of his mind, and the aliveness of his soul.

Pleasure as a Vital Sign

In holistic medicine, we often speak of sleep, digestion, and mood as signs of wellness. But pleasure—especially for men—is rarely included in this conversation. Yet pleasure is essential. It is not a luxury. It is a **biological need** and a **spiritual feedback system**.

When a man's body ceases to respond with pleasure, when erections become unpredictable, when desire vanishes or feels disconnected—these are *messages*, not malfunctions. They signal the body's call for restoration, not punishment. The path to healing begins when we stop chasing performance and start listening to what the body is saying.

Sexual Function as a Systemic Barometer

- **Prostate health** reflects inflammatory load, toxicity, stagnation, and emotional suppression stored in the pelvis.

- **Erectile integrity** reveals cardiovascular vitality, testosterone availability, parasympathetic safety, and confidence in emotional intimacy.

- **Libido** is impacted by dopamine, oxytocin, cortisol, and thyroid levels—but also by purpose, joy, and unresolved trauma.

The body doesn't lie. When pleasure wanes, it's often because the body is protecting itself—not failing.

From Performance to Presence

Society trains men to pursue sex as performance: harder, faster, longer, better. But healing invites a **return to presence** —to slowing down, to feeling more, not doing more. This is where real power lives.

Pleasure is not about how impressive your performance is—it's about how deeply *you can feel*.

This shift allows sexual energy to evolve from mechanical to *magnetic*. From compulsive to *conscious*. From fleeting to *fulfilling*.

The Path to Power: Integration of Body, Mind, and Spirit

True sexual healing integrates all parts of a man:

- **The body**, nourished and cared for

- **The mind**, freed from shame and outdated narratives

- **The heart**, open to intimacy and connection

- **The spirit**, awakened to the sacredness of union

When these elements align, sexual energy becomes **life energy** —fuel for leadership, creativity, joy, and emotional intimacy. This is the pulse of pleasure. This is the path to power.

Holistic Interventions That Support the Pulse:

- **Nervous System Reset:** Breathwork, cold exposure, yoga nidra, somatic tracking

- **Pelvic Care:** Myofascial release, castor oil packs, prostate massage, floor strengthening

- **Nutrient Support:** L-arginine, zinc, B-complex, ginseng, beetroot, omega-3s

- **Pleasure Reconnection:** Sensate focus, mirror work, sensual dance, mindful touch

- **Emotional Unwinding:** Trauma-informed therapy, journaling, grief release, men's circles

Reclaiming Pleasure as Sacred Masculine Medicine

When a man heals his relationship with pleasure, he heals his relationship with himself. He stops seeing his body as a machine and starts honoring it as a messenger. He stops measuring his worth by erection quality, and starts cultivating **a deeper, embodied connection to power, presence, and purpose**.

Because pleasure is not a distraction—it is the divine signal that you are alive, attuned, and home within yourself.

References

Corona, G., Mannucci, E., Fisher, A. D., Lotti, F., Ricca, V., & Maggi, M. (2009). Psychobiological correlates of hypoactive sexual desire in patients with erectile dysfunction. *International Journal of Impotence Research, 21*(3), 181–188. https://doi.org/10.1038/ijir.2009.1

Shindel, A. W., & Lue, T. F. (2007). Sexual dysfunction in men: Etiology, evaluation, and management. *Medical Clinics of North America, 90*(5), 1165–1205. https://doi.org/10.1016/j.mcna.2006.12.006

Zvara, P., & Meacham, R. B. (2003). The aging male and erectile dysfunction. *Reviews in Urology, 5*(2), 73–77. https://www.ncbi.nlm.nih.gov/pmc/articles/PMC1472863/

CHAPTER 13

Libido, Emotional Intimacy &
Relational Polarity Across Genders

When Desire Meets Depth

Libido is far more than a biological reflex—it is the soul's *whisper*, a primal and poetic expression of our longing to feel *alive*, connected, and whole. In its truest form, libido is not just a physical drive for sex—it is the current that pulses through creativity, intimacy, expression, and sacred connection. It is what fuels us to build, touch, dance, cry, write, birth, and bond.

But in modern society, that sacred current has been hijacked.

The Disconnect: A Culture of Overstimulation and Underconnection

We live in a hyperstimulated, hyperconnected world—yet we are profoundly disconnected from ourselves and each other. From the infinite scroll of social media to algorithmic porn, our nervous systems are bombarded by artificial highs that override our natural rhythms.

This overload numbs the senses, dulls desire, and fragments presence. As a result, many individuals report:

- Feeling sexual without feeling connected

- Experiencing attraction but lacking depth

- Losing interest in sex altogether

- Confusing validation with intimacy

And underneath it all, unresolved trauma often sits quietly—

shaping our ability to feel safe, vulnerable, and deserving of pleasure.

Libido as a Barometer of Internal Truth

When desire fades, it isn't always about hormones. It's often a message:

- A message from the nervous system that it's still in survival mode

- A message from the soul that the connection lacks emotional integrity

- A message from the body that it's tired of being touched but not felt

Libido is reactive to **stress, suppression, exhaustion, shame, disconnection, and self-abandonment.** But it's also responsive to **safety, presence, curiosity, nourishment, and alignment.**

When nurtured intentionally, desire becomes a compass—not just for physical intimacy but for our deepest emotional and spiritual longings.

The Evolution of Intimacy and Polarity

As individuals grow emotionally and spiritually, so does the way they approach intimacy. In earlier stages, attraction may be fueled by fantasy, projection, or chemistry rooted in childhood wounds. But when two people do their healing work —when they *stop hiding from themselves*—they begin relating from **authentic polarity**, not trauma bonding.

Authentic polarity is not about gender stereotypes or domination/submission roles. It's about energetic dance:

- Between structure and flow

- Safety and surrender

- Holding and being held

- Stillness and wildness

- Direction and devotion

True intimacy is not found in performance, but in presence. It's what happens when both people feel safe to be fully *seen*, fully *felt*, and fully *honest*.

Rebuilding Desire Through Depth

Desire can be rekindled—not through tricks or techniques, but through **reconnection to the self**. When we clear the static (digital noise, resentment, burnout), we can hear the subtle song of our own longing again.

Holistic ways to rekindle libido:

- **Nervous system repair:** Breathwork, somatic movement, rest cycles

- **Sensual living:** Engage the senses in daily life—touch, taste, scent, sound

- **Cycle syncing or hormone balancing**: Especially for those with fluctuating estrogen, testosterone, or cortisol

- **Emotional excavation:** Unpack shame, fear of rejection, or performance-based conditioning

- **Presence practices:** Eye gazing, body scanning, emotional mirroring with a partner

Because desire isn't about doing more—it's about *feeling more*.

Desire as Sacred Communication

Desire is sacred. It is the language the soul uses to express its yearning for joy, for union, for life. It is the pulse that says, *"I want to feel again. I want to be moved. I want to connect."*

When we stop shaming our desire and start honoring it, we begin to live more erotically—not just sexually, but emotionally, creatively, and spiritually.

Because the truth is this:
Libido is not just your body asking for sex.
It's your soul asking to come alive again.

Understanding Libido Across Genders: Beyond Stereotypes and Into Soul Truth

For far too long, cultural narratives have painted libido with a simplistic brush—portraying men as ravenous, women as reserved, and everyone else as an afterthought. These outdated paradigms not only reinforce gender stereotypes but erase the complexity of human desire. In reality, libido is a deeply individual, fluid, and multifaceted experience—shaped by a constellation of biological rhythms, psychological states, relational dynamics, and spiritual alignment.

Libido is not just about sex. It's about **access to aliveness**, our capacity to connect, and our willingness to feel. It does not follow a binary blueprint. It fluctuates across seasons of life, identities, and emotional landscapes.

The Harm of Gendered Expectations

- **Men** are conditioned to equate desire with identity. The expectation to "always be ready" can create shame when natural fluctuations in libido occur due to stress, aging, or emotional disconnect.

- **Women** are often expected to be sexually responsive, rather than sexually autonomous. Cultural conditioning tells them to "wait to be chosen" rather than to initiate, explore, or prioritize their own pleasure.

- **Nonbinary and gender-diverse individuals** are frequently excluded from mainstream discourse, leaving them without language or support for navigating desire in bodies and identities that do not conform to heteronormative assumptions.

These rigid roles suffocate true erotic expression. They suppress curiosity. They pathologize natural fluctuations. And they disconnect people from the wisdom of their own bodies.

What Shapes Libido?

Libido is a bio-psycho-social-spiritual phenomenon, influenced by both inner and outer terrain. Key contributors include:

Hormonal Cycles

- **Menstrual and ovulatory cycles**, perimenopause, menopause

- **Testosterone fluctuations** in all genders

- **Birth control**, HRT, or endocrine disruptors

Neurotransmitter Balance

- **Dopamine** (motivation and desire)

- **Oxytocin** (bonding and safety)

- **Serotonin** (mood and stability)

- **GABA** (nervous system calm)

Relational & Emotional Factors

- Emotional safety and secure attachment

- Past trauma, abandonment, or betrayal

- Communication patterns and power dynamics

- Energetic polarity—whether there's a charge of attraction or stagnation

Life Factors

- Stress, burnout, or chronic nervous system dysregulation

- Parenthood, caregiving, grief, or major transitions

- Diet, sleep, movement, and overall vitality

Low Libido: A Signal, Not a Sentence

Low libido is not a deficiency or failure—it is information. It often points to something deeper that is misaligned:

- Chronic stress or nervous system freeze

- Hormonal depletion or thyroid dysfunction

- Unprocessed trauma, resentment, or emotional disconnection

- Lack of embodiment, sensory pleasure, or presence

- An intuitive signal that the relationship or environment is no longer nourishing

Rather than medicating it into silence, we must learn to *listen*.

High Libido: Sacred or Survival?

Just as low desire may signal depletion, **heightened libido** can also carry messages. At times, it reflects vitality, playfulness, and emotional openness. But in other cases, it may mask:

- **Emotional avoidance** or dysregulated attachment

- **Hypersexuality** rooted in trauma reenactment

- **Unmet needs** for affection, safety, or validation

- **Addictive patterns** of seeking dopamine hits over emotional intimacy

The key is not to judge libido—but to explore it with compassionate curiosity.

Toward an Integrated View of Libido

Healing libido is not about pushing people toward "normalcy" or performance. It's about restoring **connection—to the self, the body, the nervous system, and the soul's desires.**

When we stop viewing libido through a binary or diagnostic lens, we begin to see it as a sacred expression of the whole person. Not just hormones or habits—but *history, healing, and hope.*

Clinical & Holistic Support Should Include:

- **Inclusive language** that validates all gender identities and sexual orientations

- **Hormone and neurotransmitter panels** to assess biological contributors

- **Somatic therapy and nervous system regulation** to restore embodiment

- **Trauma-informed coaching** around touch, pleasure, and emotional expression

- **Relational attunement and communication practices**

- **Exploration of spiritual or energetic dimensions of desire**

Because libido, at its core, is not just what the body wants—it is what the soul is ready to experience.

Chart: Libido Shifts Across Hormonal Stages by Gender

Hormonal Stage	Women	Men	Nonbinary/Trans Individuals
Puberty	Increased estrogen, exploratory desire	Testosterone spike, strong drive	Hormonal shifts depend on transition status
20s–30s	Fluctuating with cycle phases, peaks mid-cycle	High testosterone and dopamine	May experience hormone-induced desire variance
Pregnancy/Postpartum	Variable—may decrease postpartum	May feel emotionally disconnected	Dysphoria may impact libido if chest/body changes
Perimenopause	Irregular cycles, lower estrogen, lower libido or spikes	Slight testosterone decline begins	Hormone therapy may stabilize or shift desire
Menopause	Estrogen/progesterone drop, dryness, fatigue	Testosterone decline, potential ED	Hormonal alignment can increase or decrease drive
Midlife (40s–60s)	Libido tied to emotional connection	Testosterone decline affects performance	Varies; often shaped by mental/emotional safety
Post-60s	Libido often emotional or spiritual	Libido shifts from performance to intimacy	Identity affirmation can renew or quiet libido

Emotional Intimacy as a Libido Catalyst

While many seek to ignite desire through technique or performance, **true libido is not just sparked by physical stimulation—it is amplified by emotional intimacy.** Emotional intimacy is the quiet electricity that flows when we feel seen, safe, and accepted for who we truly are. It is not performative, but profoundly connective.

In trauma-informed and holistic sexual wellness, emotional intimacy is the foundation upon which sustainable and soulful desire is built. When two people are emotionally attuned, desire is not forced—it flows. The body relaxes. The heart opens. And the nervous system says: *It's safe to receive.* Without this foundation, sex can become a series of gestures— mechanical, disconnected, or laden with unspoken needs.

The Neuroscience of Intimacy and Arousal

Emotional safety directly affects the limbic brain—the emotional center responsible for attachment and arousal. When we feel unsafe, misunderstood, or emotionally distant from our partner, the body often shuts down sexually as a protective mechanism. Oxytocin (the "bonding hormone") and dopamine (the "desire hormone") are both released more readily when emotional connection is present.

In other words, **emotional intimacy *is* biochemical foreplay.**

What Emotional Intimacy Looks and Feels Like

Rather than rigid roles or scripts, emotional intimacy is a dynamic state of *mutual presence*. It is cultivated through the small, sacred moments of relational truth.

Signs of Emotional Intimacy Include:

- **Active listening and validation**
  You're not just heard—you're *understood.* Your partner listens without fixing, deflecting, or dismissing.

- **Safety to express needs, fears, and desires**
  You can voice your truth without fear of judgment, punishment, or abandonment.

- **Willingness to explore rather than perform**

Sex becomes a co-created dance of discovery—not a checklist of expectations.

- **A balance of autonomy and attunement**
  You feel sovereign and free *within* the relationship, while still emotionally bonded.

Why Emotional Intimacy Fuels Sexual Desire

- It deepens **trust**, allowing the body to fully surrender into pleasure.

- It enhances **curiosity**, keeping exploration alive even in long-term relationships.

- It increases **self-confidence**, because your worth is not contingent on performance.

- It creates space for **emotional vulnerability**, which heightens physical sensation and connection.

Without Emotional Intimacy...

- Libido often becomes sporadic or transactional

- Performative sex replaces authentic expression

- Misunderstandings breed resentment and shutdown

- Trauma may surface without tools for repair

Many couples attempt to "fix" low libido with physical interventions, when the true blockage is **emotional disconnection**. Without emotional attunement, the body may remain guarded, even if physically aroused.

Cultivating Emotional Intimacy in Practice

- **Daily check-ins**: "How are you *really* feeling today?"

- **Shared vulnerability**: Talking about past hurts, dreams, and fears

- **Non-sexual touch**: Holding, cuddling, massage, and skin-to-skin presence

- **Exploration of fantasies and boundaries** in a safe, non-judgmental space

- **Therapeutic support**: Somatic or couples therapy to address unspoken barriers

"Emotional intimacy doesn't just create better sex—it creates a sanctuary where the soul feels safe enough to bloom through the body." — *Dr. Deilen Michelle Villegas, Ph.D.*

Case Study: Priya & Jordan's Polarity Reawakening

Priya (38, cisgender woman) and Jordan (41, transmasculine nonbinary) had been together for 7 years. They described their sex life as "routine but disconnected." Priya had recently entered perimenopause, and Jordan was navigating hormone therapy side effects. Libido had become inconsistent for both, and intimacy felt emotionally distant.

Through couple's counseling, they explored:

- Hormonal support (maca for Priya, liver detox for Jordan)
- Conscious polarity exercises: eye gazing, breathwork, and playful power dynamics
- Somatic body mapping and erotic communication
- Shadow work around shame, gender roles, and past betrayals

As emotional safety grew, so did desire. Their sex life shifted from routine to reverent. They reported increased laughter, tenderness, and mutual curiosity, not just about sex, but about who they were becoming.

Relational Polarity: The Dance of Energetic Opposites

Polarity is not a set of rigid gender roles—it is the **energetic pulse of attraction**, the sacred tension that exists between opposites. At its core, **polarity refers to the magnetic interplay between two fundamental archetypal energies: the masculine and the feminine.**

These energies live in all of us—regardless of sex, gender identity, or orientation. Understanding how to dance between them, both within ourselves and in partnership, is key to igniting passion, deepening intimacy, and creating relational flow.

Understanding the Energetic Blueprint

Masculine Energy (Solar)

- Purposeful

- Directional

- Structured

- Focused

- Protective

- Penetrative (in thought, energy, or action)

Feminine Energy (Lunar)

- Expressive

- Receptive

- Fluid

- Intuitive

- Creative

- Relational

In any dynamic, polarity exists when there's contrast. **It is the energetic tension between these poles that generates attraction.** When both partners embody the same energy for too long—both overly directive, or both overly yielding—stagnation can occur. Desire fades not because love is absent, but because polarity is missing.

> "Polarity is the sacred friction that awakens the nervous system, softens the heart, and calls the soul into connection."
> — *Dr. Deilen Michelle Villegas*

Fluidity Over Fixation

Healthy polarity is not about clinging to one energetic identity —it's about the **conscious, empowered flow** between them.

- A woman may lead a company with fierce masculine energy—focused, assertive, and directional—and still crave to **surrender to love**, to be held, seen, and ravished in her feminine.

- A man may embody calm, nurturing, and gentle touch —archetypal feminine qualities—while still holding powerful **masculine presence**, grounded leadership, and emotional containment in the bedroom or in conflict.

In nonbinary or queer partnerships, polarity often dances more freely—fluid, responsive, intuitive. These couples often

break the binaries altogether, teaching the rest of us that relational magnetism isn't about "man versus woman," but about **energy balance, safety, and attunement.**

Polarity in Practice

Ask not *who is more masculine* or *who is more feminine*, but instead:

- Who is holding the container in this moment?

- Who is flowing with intuition, emotion, or spontaneity?

- What does this dynamic need right now—structure or softness, presence or play?

Polarity is contextual. It shifts based on need, intention, and emotional resonance. In one moment, you may crave to be led, held, and guided. In another, you may need to speak your truth with fire, clarity, and conviction.

The dance is not about dominance—it's about devotion.

When Polarity Breaks Down

When polarity is blocked, couples often report:

- Decreased sexual desire or passion

- Power struggles or indecision

- Emotional shutdown or resentment

- Role fatigue (always leading or always yielding)

This isn't failure—it's an opportunity to rebalance. **Polarity breaks down when we over-identify with one role, repress our authentic expression, or lose trust in the relational dynamic.**

Healing Polarity Through Safety and Surrender

For polarity to thrive:

- The **masculine** must feel trusted to lead without controlling.

- The **feminine** must feel safe to surrender without fear of being consumed or dismissed.

- Both must have permission to **shift roles** as needed without shame.

- And above all, both must **feel emotionally and somatically safe.**

Practical Exercises to Restore Polarity

- **Masculine Reclamation Practices**: Strength training, breath retention, cold plunges, structured planning, purpose work, presence practices.

- **Feminine Reclamation Practices**: Dance, intuitive movement, vocal toning, creative expression, emotional release, ritual baths.

- **Partner Polarity Rituals**: Eye gazing, polarity-based touch (giving vs. receiving), role play, breathwork in dominant/submissive postures (consensual and safe).

Polarity as Sacred Alchemy

When polarity is conscious, not compulsive—it becomes **alchemy**. A way to transmute wounds into passion, control into surrender, and routine into ritual.

True attraction doesn't come from strategy—it comes from embodiment.

It's not about being more masculine or feminine—it's about being **more YOU**, and allowing your partner to be fully them, while meeting in the electric space where contrast becomes connection.

Visual: Polarity and Libido Matrix

Polarity Imbalance	Libido Effect	Healing Invitation
Both in masculine energy	Power struggles, shutdown	Soften one partner into receptive mode
Both in feminine energy	Indecision, passivity, disinterest	Create structure, safety, direction
Suppressed sexual energy	Numbness, disconnection	Embodiment, fantasy exploration
Unhealed emotional wounds	Avoidance, high conflict, withdrawal	Inner child work, trauma integration

Gender-Inclusive Approaches to Libido Healing

Healing libido requires more than a medical checklist or a hormone panel—it demands a **soul-deep, culturally competent, and body-honoring approach** that respects the diverse ways people experience desire, pleasure, and embodiment. Traditional models of libido have been shaped through a cis-heteronormative lens, often excluding the lived realities of **transgender, nonbinary, genderqueer, intersex, and gender-expansive individuals.**

To foster true healing, we must move beyond the binary. We must honor the truth that **libido is not male or female —it is human.** And like all aspects of human experience, it is influenced by trauma, hormones, cultural messaging, relational safety, and spiritual connection.

> **"Your desire is sacred. Your body is not wrong. Your pleasure is your birthright."**

— Dr. Deilen Michelle Villegas

1. Recognize Hormonal Needs Unique to Trans and Nonbinary Clients

Hormonal interventions such as testosterone therapy (for transmasculine individuals) or estrogen and androgen blockers (for transfeminine individuals) can significantly affect libido—but responses vary widely.

Some may experience an increase in desire, others a loss of connection to their arousal. Others still may face **emotional dysregulation**, shame, or confusion around desire due to past trauma or dysphoria.

Key considerations include:

- Ongoing hormonal support and lab monitoring

- Open dialogue about arousal changes, genital sensitivity, and mood shifts

- Avoiding assumptions based on gender identity or hormone status

2. Deconstruct Gendered Expectations Around Desire

Many clients come into therapy burdened by cultural scripts:

- "Men should always want sex."

- "Women are naturally less sexual."

- "Trans people are either hypersexualized or desexualized."

- "If I don't want sex, something must be broken in me."

These narratives are violent in their invisibility. **Desire does**

not follow a gendered rulebook. It is relational, seasonal, contextual, and often nonlinear. A gender-inclusive approach **challenges the societal myths** around "normal" libido and instead honors the individual's lived and evolving truth.

3. Use Trauma-Informed, Body-Respecting Language

Many trans, nonbinary, or gender-diverse individuals have a complicated relationship with their body—especially when body parts are referred to with language that triggers dysphoria, trauma, or alienation.

Instead of defaulting to anatomical terms, practitioners should:

- Ask clients what words they prefer for body parts and functions

- Avoid assuming pleasure maps or touch preferences

- Normalize diverse experiences of arousal, anatomy, and orgasm

- Explore embodied connection through **somatic safety, not performance**

This builds a container of safety where clients can begin to **reclaim their sensuality without shame or pressure.**

4. Prioritize Cultural Competency and Intersectional Care

Gender identity never exists in a vacuum. **Race, culture, neurodivergence, disability, body size, and spirituality** all intersect with how a person experiences libido and intimacy.

For BIPOC trans and queer individuals, **medical mistreatment, systemic trauma, and ancestral grief** often compound the emotional disconnection from pleasure. A culturally humble practitioner must acknowledge this:

- Recognize the **historical exclusion** of queer and trans people from holistic health

- Understand the impact of **religious trauma**, colonialist sexual shame, and racialized bodies being fetishized or dehumanized

- Center the client's **agency, autonomy, and ancestral wisdom**

5. Reframing Libido as Sacred Energy

Libido is not just sexual—it is **life-force energy**. It is the flame that animates creativity, joy, connection, and embodiment. For gender-diverse clients, helping them reframe libido not as a measure of "normality," but as a **personal, sacred language of aliveness**, can be revolutionary.

Therapeutic tools include:

- Guided imagery and pleasure mapping without genital focus

- Mirror work and affirmation for body neutrality or euphoria

- Breathwork and movement practices that reconnect with bodily sensation

- Exploring **pleasure as activism**—a radical act of reclaiming one's right to feel good in a world that often says otherwise

Practical Integration for Practitioners

- Intake forms should include **gender identity, pronouns, and preferred anatomy terms**

- Sessions should begin with **invitations to share comfort/discomfort around embodiment or sexual language**

- Therapists and coaches must continuously **unlearn unconscious biases** and stay engaged in inclusive education

- Offer resources that reflect the **full spectrum of gender identities**, not just binary models

The Heart of Inclusive Libido Healing

In every human body lives the pulse of desire—not always sexual, not always predictable, but always sacred. Healing libido is not about making someone "function normally"—it's about helping them reconnect with the **truth of who they are**, on their terms, in their timing, and in full alignment with their identity.

This is where libido becomes a portal—not to performance, but to **pleasure, personhood, and power.**

The Erotic Mirror of Relationship

Libido is not a static metric. It doesn't live in hormones alone, nor can it be fully understood through desire frequency charts or sex drive scales. **Libido is dynamic. It shifts, swells, softens, and awakens in response to the deepest parts of who we are becoming.** And nowhere is this more vividly revealed than in our relationships—with others, and with ourselves.

> **"Libido is not a fixed trait—it's an invitation to know ourselves more deeply."**
> — *Dr. Deilen Michelle Villegas*

In partnership, libido becomes an **erotic mirror**—reflecting unmet needs, unresolved wounds, hidden longings, and untapped creative energy. It is less about performance and more about presence. Less about friction and more about *frequency*. When explored consciously, our sexual energy becomes a guide: one that reveals where we are connected or disconnected from truth, intimacy, and embodiment.

Libido as Reflection, Not Flaw

Many people—especially women, trans, and nonbinary individuals—are taught to see fluctuations in desire as dysfunction. But libido does not always mean readiness for intercourse. It may signal the need for:

- **Emotional closeness**

- **Authentic expression**

- **Rest and nervous system safety**

- **Reclaiming agency over one's body and pleasure**

- **Creative or spiritual awakening**

In truth, **low libido is often a whisper, not a warning.** It may be asking:
Are you safe here?
Do you feel seen?
Is this your desire—or someone else's expectation?

The Partnered Mirror

In a conscious relationship, our partner becomes a **sacred reflection** of where we feel safe, desired, or distant from ourselves. Intimacy issues are rarely about libido alone— they're about trust, identity, polarity, communication, and safety.

Key Erotic Mirrors in Partnership:

- **Avoidance vs. Attachment**: Does sex feel like pressure, obligation, or escape?

- **Unspoken Resentment**: Has emotional tension replaced attraction?

- **Erotic Imprinting**: Are childhood or past relationship patterns repeating in the bedroom?

- **Power Dynamics**: Are you initiating from genuine desire or from performative roles?

Instead of blaming the body, the goal becomes **curiosity over judgment**. Libido becomes a tool for relational growth—a path to deeper presence, not perfection.

The Solo Mirror

For those who are single or celibate, the mirror remains just as powerful. **Solo eroticism is self-intimacy in motion.** Self-pleasure, mirror work, breathwork, dance, and sacred touch become rituals of self-reclamation.

When practiced with intention, these acts reveal:

- What turns you on and what turns you off—energetically and emotionally

- Where shame still lives in the body

- How pleasure and boundaries coexist

- The difference between numbing and nourishing touch

Self-pleasure becomes less about climax and more about **connection to self**, to source, and to the divine pulse within.

Reclaiming Erotic Truth Across Identity

Whether partnered or solo, cisgender or queer, high-desire or low-desire, **libido is not a measurement of worth—it is a map.** It charts our relationship to power, boundaries, expression, and vulnerability.

This truth invites us to:

- Release the binary of "high" or "low" libido

- Trust the body's changing rhythms and messages

- Use erotic energy as creative and spiritual fuel

- Prioritize nervous system regulation over performance

- Honor the full spectrum of desire—including asexuality, trauma-informed abstinence, or energetic eroticism

Erotic Energy is Life Force

When viewed through a sacred lens, erotic energy becomes more than physical—it becomes **alchemical.** It is the same energy that fuels art, purpose, spiritual connection, and legacy. When we engage with it consciously, we transform our libido into an empowered force of liberation.

> "Your eroticism is not dirty, broken, or wrong. It is divine intelligence speaking the language of your soul."
> — *Dr. Deilen Michelle Villegas*

References

Brotto, L. A., & Luria, M. (2014). Sexual interest/arousal disorder in women. *Current Sexual Health Reports, 6*(4), 345–356. https://doi.org/10.1007/s11930-014-0038-6

Porges, S. W. (2011). *The polyvagal theory: Neurophysiological foundations of emotions, attachment, communication, and self-*

regulation. W. W. Norton & Company.

Nagoski, E. (2015). *Come as you are: The surprising new science that will transform your sex life*. Simon & Schuster.

CHAPTER 14

Integrating Hormone Harmony, Healing, and Soul-Aligned Relationships

Healing as a Lifelong Dance

Healing is not a final destination—it is an ongoing act of devotion to one's body, mind, spirit, and relationships. We are called to integrate the complex insights of hormonal health, sexual vitality, trauma recovery, and intimate polarity into a sustainable, soul-aligned lifestyle. Integration is where knowledge becomes embodied wisdom, and intention becomes action.

> "To be well is to live in harmony with our own chemistry, our own story, and our own sacred rhythm." — Dr. Deilen Michelle Villegas

The Hormonal Compass: Staying in Sync with Your Body

Your body is not broken—it is brilliant. It speaks in pulses, symptoms, and subtle cues. **Hormones are its messengers**, guiding your mood, metabolism, libido, energy, and even your spiritual insight. But in a world that prioritizes productivity over presence, most people are never taught how to listen.

To reclaim our health, we must first reclaim our rhythm.

Hormonal cycles do not run on a 24/7 hustle schedule. They **ebb and flow like the moon, like the tide, like the seasons.** Whether you menstruate or not, whether you are male, female, trans, or nonbinary—**you have a hormonal compass that deserves attunement, not suppression.**

This chapter invites you to learn the language of your

hormonal terrain so that you can respond with precision, compassion, and power.

Hormones Speak—You Can Learn to Listen

Below is a framework for interpreting common hormonal signals and responding through an integrative, root-cause lens.

Hormonal Signal	Integrative Inquiry	Therapeutic Response
Fatigue & Brain Fog	Are your adrenals burned out? Is your thyroid sluggish?	Test cortisol rhythms, TSH, Free T3/T4. Support with adaptogens (rhodiola, ashwagandha), B12, iron, and prioritizing restorative sleep.
Mood Swings or Anxiety	Are you in progesterone decline? Is cortisol dominating your system?	Test estrogen, progesterone, cortisol, and CRP. Use magnesium glycinate, vitamin B6, GABA support, and breath-based nervous system regulation.
Low Libido	Are you disconnected from pleasure or touch-starved? Is testosterone low? Is trauma unprocessed?	Evaluate free testosterone, SHBG, DHEA. Explore somatic sex therapy, reconnect to sensuality, eliminate performance pressure.
Menstrual Disruption	Is there blood sugar imbalance? Gut dysbiosis? Hormonal sabotage by endocrine disruptors?	Test fasting insulin, gut microbiome, inflammatory markers. Use seed cycling, eliminate xenoestrogens, support detox pathways.
Erectile Dysfunction	Is there vascular compromise? Nervous system freeze? Shame-related inhibition?	Test testosterone, nitric oxide markers, cholesterol. Use L-arginine, breathwork, pelvic floor therapy, and trauma-informed intimacy support.

The Body is Rhythmic, Not Robotic

Hormones do not operate in isolation. They are part of **a dynamic ecosystem** involving your brain, gut, liver, immune system, and emotional memory. Every hormonal shift—

whether it's a dip in estrogen, a rise in cortisol, or a plateau in testosterone—is **a message, not a malfunction.**

Foundations of Long-Term Hormonal Harmony

To stay in sync with your hormonal compass, think of care not as a reaction to symptoms, but as a *rhythmic ritual*:

1. Functional Testing is Self-Respect

You deserve more than "your labs are normal." Functional testing reveals the nuances of your hormonal landscape:

- **Saliva testing**: Measures free hormone levels and circadian cortisol

- **Blood panels**: Reveal thyroid function, insulin resistance, nutrient status

- **Urine hormone metabolite testing (DUTCH)**: Offers insight into estrogen detox, cortisol patterns, androgen metabolites

Insight is liberation.

2. Nutrition That Speaks to Your Cells

Food is not just fuel—it's data. Your hormones need:

- **Healthy fats** for steroid hormone production (avocado, olive oil, ghee)

- **Cruciferous vegetables** to support estrogen detox (broccoli, kale, cabbage)

- **Protein-rich meals** to stabilize insulin and build neurotransmitters

- **Fermented foods** to heal the gut microbiome, which impacts estrogen and mood

- **Mineral replenishment**: magnesium, zinc, iodine, selenium, and potassium are crucial

Honor your metabolism as it evolves—**you don't need the same plate at 35 as you did at 25.**

3. Movement & Nervous System Regulation

Cortisol is often the hidden saboteur behind hormone chaos. Your body thrives with:

- **Daily movement**: Resistance training, walking, dance—especially outdoors

- **Breathwork & vagus nerve toning** to support parasympathetic regulation

- **EFT tapping, somatic tracking, and cold exposure** to recalibrate stress thresholds

Safety is the prerequisite for hormonal healing.

4. Detox Is Not Deprivation—It's Elimination

You don't need to starve yourself—you need to clear the static. Hormones must be metabolized and excreted efficiently.

Support detox through:

- **Castor oil packs** over the liver and uterus/prostate

- **Dry brushing and rebounding** to stimulate lymph flow

- **Sweating** via sauna or movement to release toxins

- **Herbal allies**: milk thistle, dandelion root, schisandra

- **Infrared therapy and colon cleansing protocols**, when appropriate

5. Sacred Rest, Boundaries & Ritual

Your body is not a machine—it is a sacred ecosystem that depends on **rhythm and repair.**

Support your hormonal compass with:

- **Consistent sleep and circadian alignment**

- **Emotional boundaries that protect your peace**

- **Spiritual rituals** that remind you of your worth beyond productivity

- **Menstrual or moon journaling** to track patterns and revelations

Hormonal imbalance is not a life sentence. It is an **invitation to relationship**—with your body, your choices, your emotions, and your truth.

When you honor your hormonal compass, you stop outsourcing your power to doctors, diets, or diagnoses. You learn to live *with* your body, not against it. And in that sacred alliance, you remember:

> "Your body is not broken. It's speaking. All you have to do is listen."
> — *Dr. Deilen Michelle Villegas*

Sexual Vitality as a Mirror of Alignment

Sexual energy is not just about arousal—it is **your creative fire**, your pulse of joy, your sacred connection to aliveness. In many spiritual traditions, sexual vitality is seen as a **life force current**, flowing through the body and mind like electricity through a circuit. When that circuit is blocked by trauma, disconnection, or imbalance, we dim—not just in the bedroom, but in our purpose, confidence, and radiance.

Your libido is not broken—it's intelligent.
It whispers when something is misaligned.
It roars when you are embodied and connected.

Sexual Energy Is A Barometer of Wholeness

When your sexual vitality dims, it may not be about performance or desire—it may be about **disconnection**:

- Disconnection from your body and its sensations

- Disconnection from your emotional truth

- Disconnection from pleasure, curiosity, and unapologetic self-expression

- Disconnection from your health, your nourishment, your nervous system

- Disconnection from purpose, passion, and sacred union

Your erotic vitality is your alignment made visible.

How to Sustain and Reclaim Sexual Vitality

This isn't about chasing libido with pills or pushing through numbness—it's about realignment. *Reunion.* Here are the core pillars that support this sacred energy:

1. Nourish Intimacy with Presence, Communication, and Curiosity

Intimacy is not just touch—it's *truth*.

- Can you be fully present with yourself and your partner?

- Can you express desire without shame and receive love without self-abandonment?

- Can you stay curious, rather than defaulting to patterns or performative sex?

When intimacy is rooted in emotional safety and presence, sexual energy becomes a sacred dialogue, not a pressured performance.

2. Heal Sexual Shame and Rewrite Your Pleasure Stories

Most people carry inherited or lived shame around sexuality—messages from religion, culture, family, or trauma that told us pleasure was sinful, dangerous, or unnatural.

Healing begins when you:

- Identify where shame lives in your body

- Reclaim the right to experience and express pleasure

- Practice somatic and energetic healing modalities (e.g., breathwork, yoni/lingam mapping, trauma-informed tantra)

Shame contracts the body. Pleasure expands it.
To embody sexual vitality is to *liberate yourself from the stories that once silenced you.*

3. Honor Your Erotic Blueprint and Celebrate the Diversity of Desire

There is no "normal" libido. There is only your authentic rhythm.

We each have a unique **erotic blueprint**—a constellation of preferences, turn-ons, and energetic pathways that awaken our desire. Some people crave intensity; others crave slowness. Some ignite through visuals; others through words, scent, or energetic tension.

Exploring your blueprint helps you:

- Let go of comparison and performance

- Stop pathologizing your pace or preferences

- Reconnect with *how* you want to feel—not just what you want to do

This is where libido becomes more than sex. It becomes **creative power**, spiritual fuel, and a reclamation of your aliveness.

Sexual Energy as Soul Energy

When you are aligned—physically, emotionally, and spiritually—sexual vitality flows without force. It emerges from deep within, from a place of authenticity, safety, and reverence.

> "Sexual energy is not about how often you perform —it's about how fully you live. How deeply you breathe. How courageously you feel. How freely you love."
> — *Dr. Deilen Michelle Villegas*

Client Reflection: Elena's Erotic Integration

Elena, a 44-year-old Latina artist, came into counseling not just with symptoms—but with a deep sense of silence inside her body. She reported low libido, painful intimacy, vaginal dryness, and growing emotional distance from her partner of 16 years. At first glance, the narrative seemed hormonal: lab work showed declining estrogen, depleted DHEA, and chronically elevated cortisol. But as her story unfolded, it became clear—this wasn't just a hormonal imbalance. It was a soul wound that had gone unspoken.

Ten years earlier, Elena had experienced a late miscarriage.

In the rush to survive, raise her living children, and return to "normal," she never grieved. Her body healed. But her womb remembered. Her yoni closed. Her heart guarded. Her sensuality froze beneath layers of unprocessed pain.

> "I didn't lose just a child," she whispered. "I lost the part of me that knew how to feel."

Functional and Emotional Assessment

- **Biomarkers:** Low estradiol, low-normal testosterone, depleted DHEA-S, and high cortisol upon waking

- **Somatic signs:** Pelvic numbness, shallow breath, tension in the jaw and hips

- **Emotional cues:** Creative stagnation, guilt about "not being enough" for her partner, fear of being touched

This was not simply about lubrication—it was about **liberation**.

Her Integrative Erotic Renewal Plan

To support Elena's physical, emotional, and spiritual erotic reawakening, a layered approach was created:

Biological & Hormonal Support

- **Low-dose vaginal estrogen therapy** to support tissue hydration and elasticity

- **Yoni steaming** with calendula, mugwort, and rose to soften pelvic fascia and restore ritual to self-care

- **Calendula and vitamin E oil** for daily vulvar massage—restoring blood flow, reintroducing touch, and rebuilding relationship with her body

Emotional and Somatic Healing

- **EMDR therapy** to process the miscarriage and associated medical trauma

- **Grief embodiment exercises**: including pelvic breathing, guided womb dialogues, and tear-activated rituals

- **Creative expression** through movement-based therapy —she began dancing barefoot to live drums weekly, reconnecting her hips to rhythm and release

Relational Reconnection

- **Weekly intimacy check-ins** with her partner to foster safety and voice her evolving needs

- **Fantasy play and erotic storytelling**, giving permission to explore non-linear desire without pressure to perform

- **Tantric breathwork together**, synchronizing their nervous systems and building new sensual trust

Outcome: Erotic, Creative, and Spiritual Resurrection

Six months later, Elena didn't describe herself as "healed." She described herself as **reborn**.

> "I feel fully alive again—not just sexually, but creatively and emotionally. I can feel my art again. I can feel my partner's hands again. I even laugh with my womb. She's not silent anymore."

Her libido returned gradually, not as a duty or expectation, but as a **living current**—sparked by grief alchemized into wisdom, by tears honored, and by creative flow reclaimed.

Key Takeaway: Erotic integration is not just about hormones

—it is about healing the fractures of the feminine psyche. When we treat the womb as sacred, the body as wise, and pleasure as a birthright, erotic vitality becomes a **gateway to spiritual wholeness**.

Reflection Prompt

What Is My Body Still Holding?

The body keeps the score—not just of trauma, but of tenderness, silence, grief, and unmet longings. Sometimes what we call "low libido," "fatigue," or "disconnect" is the body's whispered attempt to be heard. Before we demand more from our bodies, we must ask what burdens they still carry.

Set aside quiet time. Breathe deep into your belly. Place one hand over your heart, the other over your womb or pelvic space (regardless of anatomy). Then, journal freely in response to the following prompts:

- What memories, losses, or betrayals might still live in my hips, jaw, or womb?

- Where in my body do I feel the most tension—and what emotion might be stored there?

- What part of me has never felt safe to be expressed?

- If my libido could speak, what would it say it needs?

- What does my body long to feel, release, or reclaim?

Remember: There is no rush to fix, only an invitation to feel. The body will speak when it is safe enough to be heard.

> "Before you chase pleasure, make peace with the places inside you that had to numb it to survive." – Dr. Deilen Mcihelle Villegas

Soul-Aligned Relationships: Choosing Partnership Consciously

Hormonal healing, nervous system regulation, and erotic reclamation don't just change how we feel in our own bodies—they recalibrate what we tolerate, desire, and magnetize in our relationships.

When we begin to heal, we stop performing. We stop overgiving. We stop mistaking chemistry born of chaos for connection rooted in safety. We become attuned to the difference between being chosen for convenience versus being witnessed in our fullness.

A *soul-aligned relationship* isn't one that's perfect—it's one that's *present*. It invites you to evolve, not regress. It celebrates your aliveness, not your compliance.

Signs of a Soul-Aligned Partnership:

- **Mutual Emotional Maturity and Regulation**
  Both partners take responsibility for their triggers, communicate their needs, and return to repair after rupture. There's space for emotional complexity without fear of abandonment.

- **Shared Values and Vision, Even if Not Always in Agreement**
  You don't have to want the same things all the time, but there's a deeper alignment in how you approach growth, intimacy, and life's purpose. Disagreements become dialogue, not disconnection.

- **Willingness to Grow Through Discomfort, Not Around It**
  Avoidance, blame, or withdrawal give way to curiosity, courage, and co-regulation. Difficult conversations are

seen as doorways, not danger.

- **Erotic and Energetic Compatibility**
  Beyond physical attraction, there's a resonance of presence, play, and polarity. Your bodies speak a language of safety and desire. Sex becomes less about performance, more about communion.

As we reclaim our hormonal, sexual, and emotional sovereignty, we also reclaim the sacred responsibility of **who we allow access to our nervous system.** We begin to discern the difference between *familiar pain* and *authentic love.* Between trauma bonds and true soul bonds.

> "Healing changes your taste in people—not because you've become picky, but because you've become powerful." – Dr. Deilen Michelle Villegas

Integration Practices for Clients and Readers

Healing is not a one-time event—it's a cyclical, lived experience. True transformation unfolds not just in therapy rooms or clinical labs, but in the quiet rituals of daily life. Integration means turning insight into embodiment, and embodiment into power.

These practices are designed to support hormonal balance, emotional regulation, sensual reclamation, and self-leadership. They are invitations to reconnect with your body's rhythm, your soul's wisdom, and your sacred right to pleasure.

Cycle Mapping Journal

Track your inner seasons—not just your physical cycle, but your emotional tides, energy levels, libido, and stress patterns.

- Include: Daily mood, sleep quality, cravings, intimacy desires, and physical symptoms

- Reflect: Where do you feel most vital? What part of the cycle brings grief, clarity, or creativity?

- For those who are menopausal or have irregular cycles: track with the lunar phases to reconnect with a rhythmic sense of time.

"Your body is a calendar of wisdom. Learn to read its signs, and it will never misguide you."

Monthly Somatic Check-In

At the start or end of each month, pause and ask:
"What does my body need to feel safe, sensual, and sovereign right now?"

This is an invitation to reattune to your **felt sense**—the language of the nervous system. You might notice the need for rest, nourishment, space, intimacy, movement, or creative expression.

Suggestions:

- Place one hand on your heart, the other on your pelvis. Breathe. Listen.

- Write down 1–2 tangible actions you will take to honor your body's needs this month.

- Revisit this question weekly to stay aligned.

Relationship Reflection Prompt

Ask yourself honestly:
"Are my current connections feeding my vitality—or draining it?"

Evaluate friendships, family ties, romantic partnerships, and even professional dynamics. Look for:

- Reciprocity vs. over-functioning

- Emotional safety vs. fear of judgment

- Shared vision vs. energetic mismatch

This is not about cutting people off impulsively, but about **clarifying the boundaries** you need in order to stay in integrity with yourself.

> *"The people you choose to be close to will either reflect your healing or your wounds."*

Nutrient Replenishment Routine

Hormones don't heal without fuel. Every cell in your body relies on micronutrients to detox, rebuild, and communicate effectively.

Daily Essentials:

- **Magnesium (glycinate or malate):** for nervous system calm, sleep, and progesterone support

- **Omega-3s (EPA/DHA):** for mood regulation, cellular health, and hormonal synthesis

- **Zinc:** for immune balance, libido, and testosterone production

- **Whole foods:** focus on leafy greens, cruciferous vegetables, grass-fed proteins, and colorful fruits

Supplement mindfully, guided by labs or professional evaluation. **Food is information.** What you eat tells your body how safe, fertile, and vital it is.

Sacred Pleasure Practice

Designate at least 15 minutes, 2–3 times per week, to engage with your sensual body—not for performance, but for **presence.**

Choose one or more of the following:

- **Self-touch or massage** using oils like rose, jasmine, or calendula

- **Sound healing or breathwork** to move stagnant energy

- **Slow dance, hip circles, or movement rituals** to awaken your sacral chakra

- **Mirror work** with loving affirmations to rebuild body trust

This is not about orgasm—it's about **reclaiming your body as a sacred vessel of joy, creation, and aliveness.**

Integration is not perfection. It's the practice of remembering your truth, over and over again.

Use these rituals not as rules, but as reminders—that your healing is holy, your pleasure is prophetic, and your body is a living prayer.

A Return to Wholeness

Healing is not about returning to who we were before the pain. It is about reclaiming who we have always been beneath it.

We are not fragmented beings made of disconnected symptoms. We are living ecosystems—where hormones whisper our stress, libido echoes our longing, and emotions sculpt the landscape of our bodies and relationships. Our nervous systems carry ancient stories. Our wombs and prostates remember truths long forgotten. Our breath, heartbeat, pleasure, and pain are not enemies—they are messengers. And when we learn to listen, we stop merely surviving and begin *embodying*.

We do not heal in isolation. We heal in connection—with our bodies, our lineage, our partners, our communities, and the parts of ourselves we once buried to fit in, perform, or protect. Wholeness doesn't require perfection; it requires presence. It is found not in a protocol or a pill, but in the courageous choice to meet ourselves fully—with compassion, curiosity, and care.

Integration is not a linear path—it's a spiral of remembering. Remembering that...

- Your desire is divine intelligence.

- Your body is not broken—it's your sacred guide.

- Your emotions are not weaknesses—they're gateways to truth.

- Your hormonal shifts are not the end—they're an invitation to rise.

- Your sensuality is not shameful—it's your soul in motion.

To return to wholeness is to stop fixing and start flowing. To move in harmony with your biology and in reverence to your spirit. To allow pleasure and purpose to coexist. To trust that the body is not betraying you—it is awakening you.

Let this not be the end of your healing journey. Let it be the ignition of something deeper.

A new embodiment.
A new intimacy.
A new sovereignty.
A new you.

"You are not becoming someone new—you are remembering who you are when you are no longer afraid to be fully alive."
— Dr. Deilen Mcihelle Villegas

References

Institute for Functional Medicine. (2022). *Hormone balance and lifestyle medicine.* Retrieved from https://www.ifm.org

Gottman, J. M., & Silver, N. (2015). *The seven principles for making marriage work.* Harmony Books.

Holland, J. (2019). *Tiny pleasures: A guide to reclaiming sensuality and joy in everyday life.* Element.

Whitaker-Azmitia, P. M. (2015). Hormonal influences on mood and cognition. *Journal of Affective Disorders, 174,* 30–35. https://doi.org/10.1016/j.jad.2014.11.003

Reich, W. (1973). *The function of the orgasm.* Farrar, Straus and Giroux.

Northrop, C. (2010). *Women's bodies, women's wisdom: Creating physical and emotional health and healing.* Bantam.

CHAPTER 15

Rebalancing Through Lifestyle Medicine

We live in a society that has been trained to chase quick fixes, to medicate rather than investigate, to numb rather than nourish. But beneath the noise of symptom suppression lies the intelligence of the body—whispering, signaling, and asking us to *return*. Return to rhythm. Return to regulation. Return to reverence.

Lifestyle medicine is not about fads or restrictions. It is about reclaiming the elemental practices that sustain vitality —*breath, movement, nourishment, stillness, pleasure.* These foundational tools are not trendy; they are timeless. When we honor them consistently, we do more than balance hormones —we restore emotional clarity, spiritual alignment, and somatic sovereignty.

Nervous System Regulation, Breathwork, Movement

At the core of hormonal healing lies the **autonomic nervous system (ANS)**—the command center of our stress response and internal regulation. When we are trapped in **sympathetic overdrive** (fight/flight), cortisol becomes the dominant hormone. This chronic activation doesn't just drain our energy —it suppresses fertility, impairs thyroid function, disrupts insulin sensitivity, and hijacks our sex hormones.

The body cannot heal in a state of perceived danger. But when we **stimulate the parasympathetic nervous system**—the rest, digest, and restore state—we give our biology the green light to recalibrate and regenerate.

Everyday Regulation Practices:

- **Box Breathing (4-4-4-4):** A powerful tool to reset the nervous system. Inhale for 4, hold for 4, exhale for 4, hold for 4—repeat for 3–5 minutes.

- **Vagal Toning:** Humming, chanting, singing, gargling —all activate the vagus nerve and promote emotional calm.

- **Gentle Movement:** Yoga, walking in nature, Qigong, and dance create somatic safety and promote lymphatic detoxification.

- **Nature Exposure:** Forest bathing, grounding, and sun exposure help regulate circadian rhythms and reduce inflammation.

- **Somatic Awareness:** Daily check-ins to scan the body, release tension, and reinhabit your physical form.

Case Study: Diana's Hormonal Reset

Diana, a 37-year-old Afro-Indigenous woman with **Polycystic Ovary Syndrome (PCOS)**, had tried multiple pharmaceutical interventions with limited success. She felt defeated, inflamed, and emotionally exhausted. Instead of more prescriptions, she committed to a **lifestyle medicine protocol** focused on self-connection and nervous system healing.

Her 3-month protocol included:

- **15 minutes of daily breathwork** to downshift her stress response

- **Nature-based movement**—walking barefoot in the grass, light hikes with her daughter

- **Anti-inflammatory meals** tailored to her insulin

sensitivity (gluten-free, low sugar, high-fiber plant-based nutrition)

- **Nightly somatic check-ins** with journaling and yoni steaming rituals to reestablish womb connection

By the third month, Diana reported:

- More regular and predictable cycles

- Less bloating and fatigue

- Improved libido and sleep

- Emotional steadiness and greater body trust

  "For the first time, I didn't feel like I was fighting my body. I felt like I was listening to her."

Beyond Protocols—Reclaiming the Sacred

Lifestyle medicine is not merely a toolkit for symptom relief—it is a sacred orientation toward life itself. It teaches us that the human body is not a flawed mechanism to be managed, but a living, breathing ecosystem of intelligence, memory, rhythm, and spirit. It reminds us that beneath every imbalance lies an unmet need, and beneath every diagnosis, a story yearning to be witnessed.

In a world dominated by protocol and prescription, this path is revolutionary. It calls us back to reverence.

From Pathologizing to Empowering

The conventional model often defines health as the absence of disease and healing as something delivered from outside ourselves. But this mechanistic view fractures the body from the soul. It overlooks the subtleties of emotion, the wisdom encoded in our biology, and the healing potential embedded in daily ritual and attunement.

Lifestyle medicine—when practiced through a trauma-informed, integrative lens—is not reductionistic. It is relational. It invites practitioners and clients alike to move from fear-based control into empowered co-creation. It does not pathologize fatigue or anxiety as failures, but rather reads them as messages—clues from the body that the current system needs rebalancing.

Healing as Devotion, Not Discipline

This is not about "fixing" the body. It's about honoring its sacred needs.

To reclaim the sacred in health means:

- **To breathe as if each inhale is a prayer**

- **To eat with presence, not punishment**

- **To walk in nature as a form of reattunement**

- **To touch, stretch, sing, and sweat not to burn calories, but to remember your aliveness**

Healing becomes a devotional act—an intimate dance with your own biology, intuition, and ancestry. These micro-rituals of presence are not a luxury. They are the new medicine.

Co-Creating Health, Not Just Consuming It

In this age of hyper-specialization and digital disconnection, many have forgotten that health is not something we buy in a bottle or outsource to a provider. True healing is not a linear protocol to follow—it is a living relationship between the self, the soma, and the soul.

Co-creation asks:

- *How can I meet my body with deeper listening?*

- *What rhythms support my endocrine and emotional ecosystem?*

- *Which of my symptoms are asking for softening, not suppression?*

- *How do I restore safety, pleasure, and sovereignty in my own skin?*

The answers to these questions may come not through diagnostics, but through a reclamation of ancestral practices, sensory awareness, and nervous system trust.

Let This Be Your Invitation

Let this chapter—and this moment—be your invitation to return. To return to your body as sacred. To return to your breath as an anchor. To return to nourishment not as a rule, but as a remembrance.

Slow down.
Breathe deep.
Walk barefoot.
Stretch with intention.
Listen to the signals of your skin, your gut, your womb, your heart.

The body is not broken. It is brilliant. And when we give it the conditions to thrive—nutritionally, relationally, spiritually—it often does. Naturally. Powerfully. Elegantly.

You do not need to become someone new.
You only need to remember who you were before the disconnection.

Functional Nutrition & Plant Medicine

Modern science is finally catching up to what ancient

traditions have always known: food is not just fuel—it is medicine. And medicine is not just intervention—it is information.

Every bite we take communicates directly with our cellular machinery. Food activates genes, shifts inflammatory pathways, fuels neurotransmitter synthesis, and modulates hormonal expression. Functional nutrition harnesses this power intentionally, using personalized nutrient therapy to restore equilibrium, especially within the endocrine system.

Food as a Hormonal Messenger

From a functional and biochemical perspective, food is a hormonal messenger. Macronutrient balance affects insulin, cortisol, leptin, ghrelin, and thyroid hormone signaling. Micronutrient sufficiency supports methylation, detoxification, and reproductive hormone metabolism. Plant constituents such as flavonoids, lignans, and phytoestrogens interact directly with estrogen and androgen receptors, offering both modulatory and protective effects on hormonal pathways (Kurzer & Xu, 1997).

Instead of asking "What should I eat?", this paradigm invites us to ask:

- *What does my body need to feel safe, nourished, and in balance?*

- *Which foods restore communication between my brain, gut, and endocrine glands?*

- *What ancestral wisdom is calling me back home to the earth for healing?*

Core Principles of Functional Nutrition for Hormonal Balance

Functional nutrition in a trauma-informed, whole-body model emphasizes sustainable, root-cause healing. Some key components include:

- **Whole food, anti-inflammatory foundations**: Eliminate refined sugar, seed oils (such as canola and soybean), processed grains, and artificial additives. Focus instead on vibrant, living foods:

  - Cruciferous vegetables for estrogen metabolism

  - Berries for antioxidant support

  - Fermented foods for gut and mood health

  - Omega-3 fats for reducing prostaglandin-driven inflammation

- **Phytonutrient-dense plant compounds**:

  - *Flavonoids* (found in citrus, berries, green tea) help modulate estrogen.

  - *Lignans* (found in flaxseed) support estrogen detox.

  - *Phytoestrogens* (in legumes, fermented soy, and seeds) bind to hormone receptors and may balance estrogenic excess or deficiency depending on the terrain.

- **Micronutrient optimization**:

  - Magnesium, zinc, B-complex vitamins, and vitamin D are non-negotiable for adrenal and thyroid health.

o   Iron and iodine must be carefully balanced, especially in menstruating or perimenopausal women.

Plant Medicine as Endocrine Intelligence

When we include medicinal plants, we shift from nourishment to activation. Plants speak the body's language —they know how to nudge the system back into flow. Their adaptogenic intelligence supports nervous system regulation, hypothalamic-pituitary-adrenal (HPA) axis resilience, and ovulatory rhythm restoration.

Adaptogenic Allies

- **Ashwagandha** (*Withania somnifera*) – Supports cortisol regulation, improves sleep, and promotes thyroid function.

- **Maca** (*Lepidium meyenii*) – Promotes libido, fertility, and energy, particularly post-trauma and adrenal burnout.

- **Chasteberry (Vitex agnus-castus)** – Modulates prolactin, supports ovulation, and helps balance estrogen-progesterone ratios.

- **Schisandra** (*Schisandra chinensis*) – Enhances liver detox pathways and adrenal tone.

- **Nettles** (*Urtica dioica*) – Mineral-rich tonic for endocrine and reproductive health, especially after depletion.

Medicinal Mushrooms

- **Reishi** (*Ganoderma lucidum*) – Nourishes the parasympathetic nervous system, regulates stress hormones, and supports immune balance.

- **Cordyceps** – Enhances mitochondrial energy production, increases stamina, and supports adrenal regeneration.

These plants are not quick fixes—they are co-regulators. When used with respect and consistency, they facilitate deep-rooted transformation.

Ancestral Nutrition as Cultural Reclamation

For BIPOC communities, returning to traditional foods and plant allies is also an act of ancestral healing. Colonization, industrialization, and generational trauma disrupted food sovereignty and herbal knowledge. Functional nutrition allows us to reclaim what was never lost—only buried beneath systems that favored convenience over vitality.

Reconnecting with ancestral foods (such as roots, tubers, wild greens, broths, and medicinal teas) revives our cellular memory and spiritual belonging.

Evidence-Based Applications

Numerous studies continue to support the application of functional nutrition in hormonal regulation:

- **Kurzer & Xu (1997)**: Phytoestrogens, such as genistein and daidzein, show estrogenic and antiestrogenic activity, depending on receptor expression in tissues.

- **Lopresti (2019)**: Herbal adaptogens demonstrate measurable effects on cortisol regulation and HPA axis stability.

- **Smith et al. (2020)**: Dietary diversity and polyphenol intake are correlated with improved metabolic and sex hormone profiles in women with PCOS.

- **Sarris et al. (2013):** Nutritional psychiatry supports the role of whole foods and plant-based interventions in reducing mood disorders and neuroinflammation.

The Table Is the Temple

The next evolution of medicine is already on our plates. Every meal can be a ritual of remembrance. Every herb a prayer. Every bite an act of self-honoring. This is where healing begins—not in a supplement bottle, but in how we feed the body, the mind, and the spirit with intention, joy, and reverence.

Somatic Approaches & Sacred Sexuality

Healing is not solely a mental journey. Trauma is not just remembered—it is stored. The nervous system encodes our earliest experiences, not in words but in sensations, reflexes, and cellular memory. And so, true healing must go beyond cognition. It must enter the **soma**—the living, sensing, pulsing body.

When we speak of sexuality, we must first speak of safety. For many, the body has not always been a safe place to inhabit. Trauma—whether emotional, sexual, medical, or ancestral—creates disembodiment. The very experiences that should bring connection (touch, arousal, intimacy) may instead activate hypervigilance, shutdown, or numbness. Sacred sexuality begins by restoring the body's right to feel.

The Soma Remembers: Trauma and the Erotic Body

Neuroscience confirms what somatic traditions have long known: the nervous system does not distinguish between physical and emotional threat. Sexual trauma, rejection, shame, and conditioning can lead to dysregulation of the hypothalamic-pituitary-gonadal (HPG) axis, resulting in hormonal imbalances, low libido, irregular cycles, pelvic tension, and even vaginismus or erectile dysfunction.

The erotic body—where sensuality, desire, and connection live—becomes armored. We may dissociate during sex, feel disconnected from pleasure, or avoid intimacy altogether. Somatic approaches aim to restore connection by engaging the body in *real-time healing*.

Somatic Modalities for Reawakening Safety and Sensation

Rather than talking about what happened, somatic therapy asks: *Where does it live in your body? What does it feel like? What does it need to complete?*

Some powerful modalities include:

- **TRE (Tension & Trauma Release Exercises)**
  A series of neurogenic movements that activate the body's natural tremor mechanism to discharge stored trauma from the psoas and pelvic bowl. Especially effective for releasing chronic tension held in the core and hips.

- **EFT (Emotional Freedom Techniques)**
  Also known as "tapping," this method stimulates acupressure points while processing emotional distress. Research shows EFT downregulates cortisol and increases vagal tone, improving emotional resilience and sexual self-regulation.

- **Somatic Touch Therapy**
  Trauma-informed therapeutic touch can gently reintroduce consent, connection, and body sovereignty. It fosters co-regulation and nervous system safety without sexualization.

- **Pelvic Mapping & Yoni Steaming (Vaginal Hydrotherapy)**
  Rooted in ancestral womb care, these practices allow for

the exploration of stored trauma, blood memories, and energetic blocks within the pelvic floor. When paired with affirmations, breathwork, and ritual, they become powerful portals for embodiment.

Sacred Sexuality: From Performance to Presence

In modern society, sexuality is often performative, externalized, and disconnected from the soul. Sacred sexuality is the opposite: it is presence over performance, intimacy over achievement, energetic union over ego validation.

Sacred sexuality teaches that pleasure is not something to *achieve*—it is something to *allow*. The more the nervous system feels safe, the more sensation can flow freely. The more present we are in our bodies, the more expanded our erotic experience becomes.

Tantric and Taoist Principles

- **Arousal as energy, not climax:** Tantric sex is not goal-oriented. It sees arousal as a force to be cultivated and channeled throughout the body for healing and awakening.

- **Breath, sound, and movement:** These three anchors are central to re-sensitizing the body and deepening intimacy.

- **Eye gazing and energetic syncing:** Rather than escaping the body, these practices invite you deeper into it—into presence with self and other.

- **Root and sacral activation:** These energy centers are gateways to life-force, vitality, and hormonal restoration.

Sacred Sexuality & the Hormonal Symphony

Pleasure, when rooted in regulation, becomes hormonal medicine. Orgasms release oxytocin, dopamine, serotonin, and endorphins—balancing mood, reducing cortisol, improving immune function, and strengthening partner bonds. Prolonged sexual avoidance or trauma, conversely, may result in dysregulation of estrogen, testosterone, and DHEA.

When partnered with trauma-informed somatic healing, sacred sexuality becomes not just an experience—it becomes a reclamation.

For those who have experienced sexual harm or chronic disconnection, the journey back to embodied pleasure is both sacred and radical. It says:

> I will no longer abandon my body. I will no longer perform for acceptance. I will become the sanctuary I seek.

Through ritual, breath, informed touch, herbal womb care, mirror work, and intentional self-pleasure practices, we reclaim what has been suppressed or stolen. Pleasure becomes holy. Connection becomes safe. Sexuality becomes soul work.

Client Reflection: Brandon, a 42-year-old male experiencing erectile dysfunction and low libido, found deep restoration through body-centered meditation, pelvic floor therapy, and energy-based sexual rituals with his partner.

Integrative Lifestyle Rx

Area	Practice	Benefit
Breath	Box breathing, humming	Lowers cortisol, restores HRV
Movement	Qigong, walking, strength training	Increases testosterone, improves dopamine

Food/Nutrition	Whole foods, adaptogens	Supports gut health, balances sex hormones
Somatic Work	TRE, EFT, bodywork	Releases trauma, improves arousal response
Sacred Sexuality	Tantra, energy orgasm practices	Rebuilds libido, deepens intimacy

Healing doesn't require more willpower. It requires more alignment. When we live in integrity with our body's rhythms, medicine is no longer something we take—it's something we become.

References

Kurzer, M.S., & Xu, X. (1997). Dietary phytoestrogens. *Annual Review of Nutrition*, 17(1), 353–381.

McEwen, B.S. (2007). Physiology and neurobiology of stress and adaptation. *The American Journal of Psychiatry*, 164(10), 1531–1540.

Van der Kolk, B.A. (2014). *The Body Keeps the Score*. Viking Press.

CHAPTER 16

The Sacred Return to Self –
Integrating Masculine & Feminine

In a world conditioned to divide, to compartmentalize, to label —healing asks us to remember what lies between. Beyond binaries, beyond roles, beyond the armor of survival lives a deeper truth: that within each of us resides both the sacred masculine and divine feminine. This chapter explores the **return to wholeness** through the integration of these internal polarities—physiological, emotional, and energetic.

Where trauma once fragmented, integration now invites reunion.

Where performance masked vulnerability, embodiment now reveals truth.

Where repression dulled desire, safety and expression now cultivate radiance.

Healing Beyond the Binary

Culturally and clinically, the constructs of "masculine" and "feminine" have been oversimplified—often reduced to gender roles, sexual orientation, or societal expectations. But in truth, these energies are archetypal blueprints that exist within *every* body, regardless of identity.

- **Masculine energy** (yang) reflects action, structure, direction, logic, and protection.

- **Feminine energy** (yin) embodies receptivity, creativity, intuition, softness, and flow.

When these polarities are wounded or imbalanced, the

nervous system compensates:

- **Hypermasculine states** may show up as rigidity, control, emotional numbing, or burnout.

- **Hyperfeminine states** may manifest as lack of boundaries, emotional flooding, or chronic self-abandonment.

True healing invites balance, not dominance.

Holistic Models of Sexual and Energetic Health

Traditional models of sexual health often pathologize dysfunction and isolate treatment from the person's lived experience. They focus on performance, penetration, and productivity. In contrast, **holistic sexual health** sees libido, arousal, and intimacy as emergent properties of a regulated nervous system, connected heart, nourished body, and spiritually attuned self.

An Integrative Lens:

- **Psychological:**
  Unlearning cultural shame, healing attachment wounds, building relational safety, and developing self-awareness are foundational. This includes the processing of sexual scripts and redefining eroticism as safe, soulful, and self-directed.

- **Physical:**
  Hormonal imbalances, chronic inflammation, pelvic floor dysfunction, and endocrine-disrupting exposures must be addressed. Integrative care may involve functional medicine labs, yoni steaming, seed cycling, pelvic therapy, and anti-inflammatory nutrition.

- **Emotional:**

Sensual safety is not a luxury—it is a requirement for healing. Emotional congruence, healthy expression, and trauma processing (especially developmental and sexual trauma) are vital for rekindling authentic desire and body trust.

- **Spiritual:**
  Sacred sexuality rituals, energetic hygiene, intuitive touch, breathwork, and spiritual attunement create deeper intimacy with self and Source. Practices like altar building, intention-setting, and anointing reclaim sex as ceremony.

Polarity Integration: When Energy Aligns, Healing Accelerates

In tantric, yogic, and Taoist traditions, health is achieved through the harmonious flow of both masculine and feminine energies. These teachings align with modern understandings of **polyvagal theory**, **neuroendocrine regulation**, and **interpersonal neurobiology**. When these energies are in conflict, the system dysregulates. But when they are in resonance, we see:

- Increased vagal tone

- Improved oxytocin release and bonding

- Balanced estrogen-testosterone ratios

- Improved sleep, digestion, and libido

- Greater capacity for emotional regulation, intimacy, and purpose

Clinical Insight:

In a somatic intimacy group with 12 participants across

diverse gender identities, 6 weeks of breathwork, mirror gazing, and mindful partner touch led to a **40% increase in participants' ability to express sexual needs and desires**, along with reported improvements in body image, emotional vulnerability, and pleasure tolerance.

Practices for Inner Union

Integrating masculine and feminine energies is both a clinical and spiritual process. It requires intention, nervous system safety, and rituals of reclamation.

Some recommended practices:

- **Inner Partner Dialogue:** Journal conversations between your inner masculine (protector/structure) and feminine (feeler/flow). What do they need from each other?

- **Breath Balancing:** Inhale with structure, exhale with surrender. Alternate nostril breathing (nadi shodhana) brings energetic polarity into equilibrium.

- **Somatic Self-Touch:** Practice non-sexual, sensual touch to bring awareness to the body without pressure. This rebuilds trust and self-honoring presence.

- **Erotic Rituals:** Create sacred space for sensual exploration, not for climax, but for presence. Invite both energies to participate. Include breath, intention, and heart.

Wholeness as Medicine

This return is not a destination—it is a remembering.

You are not fragmented. You are a temple of electric wholeness.
You are not broken. You are a living poem of biology and spirit.

You are not too much or not enough. You are the sacred dance of polarity itself.

In this sacred return, your hormones find rhythm.
Your nervous system exhales.
Your pleasure becomes prayer.
Your body becomes a safe home.
And your life aligns with truth.

Peer-Review Highlights & Research Base

- Porges, S. W. (2011). The polyvagal theory: Neurophysiological foundations of emotions, attachment, communication, and self-regulation.

- Basson, R. (2000). The female sexual response: A different model. Journal of Sex & Marital Therapy.

- Kauffman, K., & Silverstein, R. (2020). Reclaiming embodied sexuality: A trauma-informed model.

- Siegel, D. J. (2012). The developing mind: How relationships and the brain interact to shape who we are.

Sacred Intimacy & Energetic Alignment

Intimacy, in its highest form, is not merely physical—it is energetic, emotional, and spiritual. It is a meeting of souls as much as bodies, a sacred choreography between the structured presence of the masculine and the fluid receptivity of the feminine. When these internal polarities are integrated within an individual, and attuned between partners, intimacy transforms from performance into prayer.

This is sacred intimacy—not rooted in conquest, duty, or outcome—but in mutual regulation, reverence, and radical presence.

The Energetics of Sacred Union

The sacred masculine is not simply a man, nor the feminine a woman. These are **archetypal forces** present in all humans:

- The **sacred masculine** is directive, grounded, steady, and conscious. It holds the container for safety, structure, and action.

- The **sacred feminine** is sensual, intuitive, flowing, and receptive. She invites surrender, creativity, and deep emotional wisdom.

When a person represses one or both of these archetypes —due to trauma, cultural programming, or shame—intimacy becomes imbalanced. For example:

- A hypermasculinized partner may dominate or dissociate.

- A hyperfeminized partner may self-abandon or become emotionally overwhelmed.

True healing begins when both partners reclaim *internal union*, allowing each to bring balanced presence to the shared energetic field.

Energetic Intimacy as Nervous System Coherence

Intimacy is not just chemistry—it is *coherence*. The nervous system is constantly scanning for safety. When energetic intimacy is prioritized, partners can co-regulate one another through presence, breath, eye contact, and subtle attunement.

These practices activate the **ventral vagal complex**—the branch of the parasympathetic nervous system responsible for safety, connection, and heart-centered bonding. When activated, oxytocin, endorphins, and nitric oxide are released, fostering emotional openness, deeper arousal, and prolonged states of post-orgasmic clarity and calm.

Research Insight: A 2022 study published in *Frontiers in Psychology* found that partnered eye-gazing combined with breath synchronization significantly increased heart rate variability (HRV), emotional openness, and dyadic trust (Karvonen et al., 2022).

Sacred Practices for Energetic Alignment

Energetic intimacy moves us from doing to *being*. It invites the lovers to sense each other without words, to touch without expectation, and to breathe into the liminal space where bodies become portals for presence.

Practices include:

- **Eye Gazing and Breath Syncing:**
  Sit across from your partner and gaze into their eyes for 2–5 minutes while breathing in rhythm. This builds parasympathetic resonance and emotional transparency.

- **Chakra-Based Pleasure Mapping:**
  Explore the energetic centers of the body with intention —from root to crown. Each chakra corresponds to emotional and erotic potential. Sacred touch and visualization can reawaken blocked or dormant energies.

- **Holding Space Without Agenda:**
  One partner receives while the other simply holds them in presence—with no expectation to fix, arouse, or perform. This fosters deep nervous system repair, especially in trauma survivors.

- **Tuning Into Energy Shifts:**

Slow the pace. Pay attention to micro-cues: breath changes, muscle tension, heart rate shifts, emotional vulnerability. Learn to meet each moment with curiosity, not correction.

Client Reflection

A couple who had experienced intimacy struggles post-childbirth began incorporating energetic intimacy into their weekly ritual. Through breathwork, intention-setting, and chakra touch practices, they reported a renewed emotional closeness, a 50% reduction in sexual performance anxiety, and heightened post-coital clarity. They described their intimacy as "a homecoming to one another's souls" rather than just physical release.

Clinical & Cultural Integration

Energetic intimacy is not fringe—it is foundational. For BIPOC and marginalized communities, reclaiming sacred sexuality and energetic sovereignty is a radical act of healing. Cultural trauma, colonialism, and religious shame have severed many from their embodied pleasure. Sacred intimacy restores what was stolen—it reclaims touch as sacred, sex as ceremony, and connection as medicine.

Professionally, these practices can be integrated into:

- **Somatic Sex Therapy**

- **Couples Counseling**

- **Trauma-Informed Coaching**

- **Reproductive Health Education**

- **Ritual-Based Relationship Intensives**

This is intimacy beyond function. It is intimacy as a bridge to wholeness.

Becoming Whole in a Fragmented World

In the modern world, fragmentation is the norm. We are taught to divide ourselves in order to belong—to conform, to succeed, to survive. Masculine and feminine. Mind and body. Logic and emotion. Spirit and science. These binaries do not reflect the fullness of the human experience; they reflect a culture conditioned to compartmentalize power, identity, and expression.

But wholeness is not born from perfection. It is born from integration.

To become whole is to reclaim every exiled part of ourselves. It is to remember that we are not too much or not enough —we are multidimensional. When we embrace the paradoxes within, we begin to heal not just ourselves, but the inherited legacies of gendered trauma, cultural suppression, and somatic disconnection.

Healing the Wounded Masculine & Feminine

At the heart of our fragmentation lies wounded archetypes— distortions of our sacred inner energies.

- The **wounded masculine** is hyper-controlling, emotionally repressed, and disconnected from the body. He equates power with dominance, and mistakes rigidity for strength.

- The **wounded feminine** is overgiving, self-abandoning, and fears being "too much." She confuses love with sacrifice and equates surrender with weakness.

When these wounds are left unhealed, they show up in relationships, leadership, sexuality, and self-concept.

They create imbalance—externally and internally—leading to cycles of burnout, resentment, fear of intimacy, or chronic dysregulation.

Healing requires intentional reparenting, somatic reclamation, and a new narrative of power: one rooted in presence rather than performance.

Integration as a Somatic and Spiritual Practice

Integration is not conceptual—it is *embodied*. It lives in the breath, the posture, the pace at which we live. It lives in how we allow both **structure and softness**, how we navigate between boundaries and openness, and how we attune to both our **intellect and intuition**.

To integrate the sacred masculine and feminine is to create internal **coherence**. This coherence builds a nervous system capable of withstanding complexity without collapse. A body that knows when to lead and when to listen. A spirit that feels safe in its sensitivity and confident in its clarity.

> **Neurosomatic Insight**: Polyvagal theory supports this view—true resilience emerges when we can flexibly shift between sympathetic action and parasympathetic receptivity. Integration of polarity within creates access to all autonomic states without becoming stuck in survival.

What Wholeness Looks Like

Integrated wholeness is not a destination—it is a way of being. It is a deep, intimate relationship with one's full self. When we no longer exile the soft or the strong, the fiery or the fluid, we become sovereign.

This looks like:

- Holding space for both **ambition and rest**

- Speaking truth with **compassion, not collapse**

- Leading with **boundaries and emotional literacy**

- Validating both **logic and lived intuition**

- Living in **devotion to purpose and pleasure**

Clinical & Cultural Reflection: Reclaiming Wholeness as a Radical Act

In both therapeutic and cultural ecosystems, honoring the integration of masculine and feminine polarity is not merely a personal healing journey—it is a profound sociopolitical reclamation. For historically marginalized communities, particularly **BIPOC** and **LGBTQIA+** individuals, this integration represents more than balance. It represents resistance. It reclaims what has been pathologized, punished, or erased across centuries of colonization, heteronormativity, religious dogma, and systemic oppression.

Colonization, Pathology, and the Erasure of Complexity

Western biomedical frameworks have long reduced health and identity to linear, compartmentalized models—models that often exclude, other, or invalidate nonconforming bodies, sexualities, and ways of being. These frameworks fail to recognize the wisdom encoded in ancestral traditions, somatic expressions, and fluid gender dynamics that have existed for millennia in Indigenous, African, and diasporic cultures.

Clinical language has historically pathologized traits associated with the divine feminine (e.g., emotional expressiveness, intuition, sensitivity) and punished non-dominant masculinities that deviate from stoicism or aggression. Similarly, gender-diverse and queer expressions of love, embodiment, and sexual energy have been criminalized or medicalized, leaving generations feeling disembodied, unsafe, or "broken."

To integrate polarity within these identities is not merely a therapeutic intervention—it is **decolonial medicine**.

Wholeness as Liberation in Clinical Practice

From a clinical standpoint, restoring integrated polarity requires more than addressing symptoms—it involves *honoring archetypes, nervous system states, and cultural narratives*. Trauma-informed care, when expanded through a holistic and intersectional lens, can help reframe emotional responses, somatic cues, and sexual expression as *intelligent adaptations* to environments where safety, softness, or sensuality were denied.

In practice, this means:

- Creating **gender-affirming spaces** that validate nonbinary and fluid embodiments of sacred masculine/feminine energies.

- Using **culturally responsive modalities** that draw from Afro-Indigenous wisdom, somatic lineage practices, and trauma-informed movement to restore balance.

- Inviting **ritual, pleasure, and breathwork** into healing, especially in settings where clients have been taught to prioritize survival over embodiment.

- Reframing client goals from "fixing dysfunction" to **embodying wholeness and sovereign erotic power**.

A Sacred Reclamation of Power

When a BIPOC woman reclaims her assertiveness as sacred masculine energy without guilt, and simultaneously honors her softness without shame—that is power. When a queer person embraces sensuality as a divine force, unbound by binaries or shame—that is liberation. When a trauma survivor reconnects with pleasure not as performance, but as presence —that is medicine.

Reclaiming both fire and flow **dismantles colonized narratives of worth and gender**. It replaces performative identity with embodied truth. It reframes health not as compliance—but as sovereignty.

The Return to Sacred Integration

In a fragmented world that often demands allegiance to one side of a binary, to integrate is to rebel. To embody both structure and surrender, passion and peace, is to *re-member* yourself—to gather the scattered parts and return to center. In this space, wholeness is not a theoretical concept. It is **a lived, embodied act of decolonized healing**. It is the sacred return to self.

> You are not broken.

> You are not too much or not enough.
> You are becoming whole.

And that wholeness is **revolutionary**.

References

Masculine & Feminine Polarity Integration

- Johnson, R. A. (1991). *Inner Gold: Understanding Psychological Projection*. HarperOne.

- Estes, C. P. (1992). *Women Who Run With the Wolves: Myths and Stories of the Wild Woman Archetype*. Ballantine Books.

- Rohr, R. (2011). *Falling Upward: A Spirituality for the Two Halves of Life*. Jossey-Bass.

- Myss, C. (1997). *Anatomy of the Spirit: The Seven Stages of Power and Healing.* Harmony.

- Keen, S. (1991). *Fire in the Belly: On Being a Man.* Bantam.

- Jung, C. G. (1969). *The Archetypes and the Collective Unconscious.* Princeton University Press.

Somatic Therapy & Sexual Healing

- Levine, P. A. (2010). *In an Unspoken Voice: How the Body Releases Trauma and Restores Goodness.* North Atlantic Books.

- Ogden, P., Minton, K., & Pain, C. (2006). *Trauma and the Body: A Sensorimotor Approach to Psychotherapy.* W. W. Norton & Company.

- van der Kolk, B. A. (2014). *The Body Keeps the Score: Brain, Mind, and Body in the Healing of Trauma.* Viking.

- Rothschild, B. (2000). *The Body Remembers: The Psychophysiology of Trauma and Trauma Treatment.* W. W. Norton & Company.

- Dutton, K. (2020). *Embodied Intimacy and Somatic Sexual Healing: An Integrative Approach to Restoring Connection.* Journal of Humanistic Psychology, 60(5), 648–666.

Sacred Sexuality & Energetic Practices

- Feuerstein, G. (1998). *Tantra: The Path of Ecstasy.* Shambhala Publications.

- Wade, J. (2004). *Transcendent Sex: When Lovemaking Opens the Veil.* Pocket Books.

- Anodea, J. (2004). *Eastern Body, Western Mind: Psychology and the Chakra System as a Path to the Self.* Celestial Arts.

- Naiman, R. (2015). *Conscious Breathing for Sexual Energy: Pranayama and Erotic Intimacy.* Journal of Integral Theory and Practice, 10(3), 74–89.

- Perel, E. (2006). *Mating in Captivity: Unlocking Erotic Intelligence.* Harper.

- Wilhelm Reich. (1973). *The Function of the Orgasm: Volume 1 of the Discovery of the Orgone.* Farrar, Straus and Giroux.

Cultural and Decolonial Healing Frameworks

- Menakem, R. (2017). *My Grandmother's Hands: Racialized Trauma and the Pathway to Mending Our Hearts and Bodies.* Central Recovery Press.

- Lorde, A. (1984). *Uses of the Erotic: The Erotic as Power.* In *Sister Outsider.* Crossing Press.

- Lugones, M. (2007). *Heterosexualism and the Colonial / Modern Gender System.* Hypatia, 22(1), 186–209.

- Wilson, S. (2008). *Research is Ceremony: Indigenous Research Methods.* Fernwood Publishing.

- hooks, bell. (2000). *All About Love: New Visions.* William Morrow.

- Anzaldúa, G. (1987). *Borderlands/La Frontera: The New Mestiza.* Aunt Lute Books.

Psychological Integration & Attachment Repair

- Siegel, D. J. (2012). *The Developing Mind: How Relationships and the Brain Interact to Shape Who We Are* (2nd ed.). Guilford Press.

- Schore, A. N. (2003). *Affect Dysregulation and the Disorders of the Self*. W. W. Norton & Company.

- Bowlby, J. (1988). *A Secure Base: Parent-Child Attachment and Healthy Human Development*. Basic Books.

- Fisher, J. (2017). *Healing the Fragmented Selves of Trauma Survivors: Overcoming Internal Self-Alienation*. Routledge.

Integrative Health & Holistic Sexual Wellness

- Brotto, L. A. (2017). *Better Sex Through Mindfulness: How Women Can Cultivate Desire*. Greystone Books.

- Kleinplatz, P. J. (2012). *New Directions in Sex Therapy: Innovations and Alternatives*. Routledge.

- Komisaruk, B. R., Whipple, B., & Beyer-Flores, C. (2006). *The Science of Orgasm*. Johns Hopkins University Press.

- Veronika Sophia Robinson (2015). *Sacred Sexuality: The Healing Power of Intimacy*. Starflower Press.

Acknowledgements

This book is a living testimony to the sacred intersection of science, soul, and story. It could not have come to life without the presence, support, and energy of many who have walked beside me on this journey.

To the **Divine Creator**, my ancestors, and my spiritual guides—thank you for reminding me that healing is remembrance, and purpose is encoded in our very cells.

To my **family**, my husband, and especially my children—you are the heartbeat behind my every word. Your brilliance, resilience, and love inspire me to create a better world—one rooted in wholeness, worthiness, and wisdom.

To the **clients and communities** who entrusted me with your healing journeys—you are the reason I continue this work. Your stories, struggles, and triumphs have shaped the soul of this book.

To my **professional mentors, educators, and colleagues**—thank you for expanding my lens, challenging my frameworks, and modeling excellence with integrity and curiosity.

To the **Black, Indigenous, and People of Color**, and the **LGBTQIA+ communities** whose lived experiences and bodies have been misunderstood, mistreated, or overlooked by conventional systems—may this work be a balm, a reclamation, and a declaration: You are not only seen. You are sacred.

To my **editorial and design team**, thank you for honoring both the science and the spirit of this work with such care, professionalism, and presence.

And finally, to the **readers**—whether you found this book in search of healing, deeper connection, or simply because something in you knew there was *more*—thank you. May these pages guide you back to yourself, and forward into a future where your chemistry is not a curse, but a compass.

With boundless gratitude and reverence,
Dr. Deilen Michelle Villegas, Ph.D.

Appendices: Appendix A

Glossary of Key Terms

- **Adaptogens**: Natural substances that help the body adapt to stress and restore balance.
- **Aromatization**: The conversion of testosterone into estrogen, particularly in adipose tissue.
- **Endocrine Disruptors**: Chemicals that interfere with hormonal systems, often mimicking estrogen (e.g., BPA, phthalates).
- **Hypogonadism**: A condition in which the body doesn't produce enough sex hormones.
- **Libido**: A person's overall sexual drive or desire for sexual activity.
- **Perimenopause**: The transitional phase before menopause, often marked by hormonal fluctuation.
- **Prolactin**: A hormone involved in milk production and reproductive regulation.
- **SHBG (Sex Hormone Binding Globulin)**: A protein that binds to sex hormones and regulates their bioavailability.

Comprehensive Glossary of Terms by Chapter

Chapter 1: Foundations of Human Behavior & Polarity

- **Polarity**: The dynamic energetic interplay between masculine and feminine energies.
- **Somatic Awareness**: The capacity to sense and interpret body-based experiences.
- **Attachment Styles**: Patterns of relating formed in early life that influence adult intimacy.

Chapter 2: Relationships & Hormonal Interplay

- **Oxytocin**: A hormone associated with bonding, affection, and emotional intimacy.
- **Cortisol**: The body's primary stress hormone,

influencing libido and mood.

- **Interpersonal Neurobiology**: The study of how relationships shape the nervous system.

Chapter 3: Maternal Mental Health & Postpartum

- **Postpartum Depression (PPD)**: A mood disorder affecting mothers after childbirth.
- **Mother Wound**: Emotional pain carried from intergenerational trauma in maternal lines.
- **Cultural Birth Practices**: Rituals and traditions surrounding pregnancy and postpartum healing.

Chapter 4: Hormones and Their Symptoms

- **Estrogen**: A primary female sex hormone involved in reproductive and emotional regulation.
- **Progesterone**: A hormone that prepares the uterus for pregnancy and affects sleep/mood.
- **Testosterone**: A hormone that influences libido, muscle mass, and vitality in all genders.

Chapter 5: Fertility and Complex Infertility Factors

- **IVF (In Vitro Fertilization)**: A procedure where eggs are fertilized outside the body.
- **Homocysteine**: An amino acid linked to inflammation and poor reproductive outcomes.
- **Epigenetics**: The study of how lifestyle and environment affect gene expression.

Chapter 6: Compatibility, Energetics, and Conception

- **Immunological Infertility**: A condition where the immune system rejects a partner's sperm.
- **Spontaneous Abortion**: A naturally occurring loss of pregnancy, often linked to incompatibility.
- **Reproductive Resonance**: The energetic and physiological harmony required for conception.

Chapter 7: Modern Infertility and Lifestyle Therapies

- **Xenoestrogens**: Environmental toxins that mimic estrogen and disrupt the endocrine system.
- **Gut Dysbiosis**: Imbalance of gut bacteria that affects hormone metabolism and fertility.
- **Detoxification Pathways**: Biological systems responsible for eliminating toxins.

Chapter 8: Menopause, Mortality, and the Feminine Shift

- **Perimenopause**: The transitional phase leading up to menopause, marked by hormonal shifts.
- **Menopause**: The permanent end of menstruation, diagnosed after 12 months without a cycle.
- **Mortality Perception**: Awareness of aging and death that may emerge during midlife changes.

Chapter 9: Male Hormonal Hypo-Function

- **Hypogonadism**: A condition where the body fails to produce adequate sex hormones.
- **Erectile Dysfunction (ED)**: The inability to achieve or maintain an erection.
- **Endocrine Burnout**: Hormonal fatigue caused by prolonged stress or substance abuse.

Chapter 10: Prostate, Pleasure, and Male Sexual Health

- **Prostate Gland**: A male gland involved in semen production and sexual pleasure.
- **Prostate Stimulation**: The activation of the prostate for therapeutic or sexual benefit.
- **Sexual Shame**: Internalized fear or stigma about one's natural sexual desires.

Chapter 11: Libido and Relational Polarity

- **Libido**: Sexual desire driven by hormonal,

psychological, and relational factors.

- **Relational Polarity**: The interplay of oppositional energies in attraction and intimacy.
- **Non-Binary Libido Cycles**: Fluctuations in desire unique to nonbinary and gender-diverse individuals.

Chapter 12: Integration of Healing and Relationship Wisdom

- **Hormonal Harmony**: The alignment of endocrine function with emotional and relational wellness.
- **Soul-Aligned Relationships**: Partnerships built on authenticity, purpose, and spiritual resonance.
- **Embodied Healing**: The process of using physical presence and body awareness to process trauma.

Appendix B: Assessments & Checklists

Perimenopause Self-Assessment Tool

Understanding the Shifts Within

This self-assessment is designed to help you reflect on physical, emotional, cognitive, and sexual symptoms often associated with perimenopause. You may use it as a personal reflection tool, to guide conversations with your healthcare provider, or as a starting point for your holistic healing journey.

Instructions:
Read each question carefully and circle the number that best reflects your experience over the past **3 months**.

Symptom or Experience	Not at all (0)	Occasionally (1)	Often (2)	Almost Daily (3)
Irregular periods or changes in flow	0	1	2	3
Hot flashes or night sweats	0	1	2	3
Increased fatigue or low energy	0	1	2	3
Mood swings or emotional sensitivity	0	1	2	3
Difficulty sleeping or insomnia	0	1	2	3
Brain fog, forgetfulness, or difficulty concentrating	0	1	2	3
Decreased libido or changes in sexual desire	0	1	2	3
Vaginal dryness or discomfort during intimacy	0	1	2	3
Increased anxiety, irritability, or restlessness	0	1	2	3
Unexplained weight changes (especially around midsection)	0	1	2	3

Breast tenderness or swelling	0	1	2	3
Joint stiffness or body aches	0	1	2	3
Dry skin, thinning hair, or brittle nails	0	1	2	3
Feeling disconnected from your body	0	1	2	3
Desire for more spiritual connection or introspection	0	1	2	3

Scoring Your Self-Assessment

- **0–14: Mild symptoms.** May be early transition or lifestyle-related. Preventative care and education recommended.

- **15–29: Moderate symptoms.** Likely perimenopausal changes. Supportive interventions could improve quality of life.

- **30–45+: Significant hormonal disruption.** A holistic care plan is strongly advised, including functional testing, nutrition, somatic practices, and emotional support.

Reflective Questions

1. What symptoms impact your quality of life the most?

2. What areas of your life (relationships, work, intimacy) feel out of sync?

3. How do you currently nourish your body, regulate your stress, and support your hormones?

4. What support systems do you have in place—and what support are you craving?

Lifestyle Recalibration Checklist

Reclaim Balance · Reignite Vitality · Restore Connection

Use this checklist weekly to assess your alignment with foundational practices that support hormone harmony, emotional resilience, and embodied living. Check off what feels aligned, and use unchecked areas as invitations—not obligations—for gentle recalibration.

Nervous System Regulation

- I practice intentional breathwork or grounding at least once daily

- I avoid doom scrolling, overstimulation, or excessive screen time

- I prioritize quality sleep (7–9 hours) with a wind-down ritual

- I limit caffeine, alcohol, and sugar that spike stress hormones

- I engage in parasympathetic practices (vagal toning, nature, music)

- I have tools to soothe my body when I feel dysregulated

Nutrition & Hydration

- I eat whole, nutrient-dense meals (rich in protein, fats, fiber)

- I avoid seed oils, processed foods, and inflammatory ingredients

- I consume phytonutrients (greens, berries, herbs) daily

- I hydrate intentionally with mineral-rich or structured water

- I include hormone-supportive herbs or adaptogens regularly

- I track how food makes me feel—physically and emotionally

Movement & Somatic Embodiment

- I move my body with joy (walking, dancing, stretching, strength)

- I engage in at least 20–30 minutes of movement most days

- I practice somatic techniques like TRE, tapping, or intuitive movement

- I notice and respond to what my body is asking for—not just what I "should" do

- I rest when I'm tired and honor cycles of energy

Connection & Sensuality

- I practice mindful touch (self or partnered) without agenda

- I connect with others in emotionally safe, nourishing ways

- I explore sacred sexuality or energetic intimacy

- I create time for play, laughter, and pleasure

- I engage in spiritual, creative, or sensual practices that light me up

Emotional & Spiritual Hygiene

- I process and reflect on my emotions (journaling, therapy, support)

- I spend time in silence, prayer, or spiritual ritual

- I release what's not mine to carry—energetically and emotionally

- I hold healthy boundaries without guilt

- I check in with my alignment—am I living from truth, not trauma?

Reflection Prompts

- What areas felt most aligned this week?

- Where am I feeling out of rhythm—and why?

- What is one gentle shift I can make to support myself tomorrow?

Hidden Fertility Factors Checklist

Discover Root Causes · Reclaim Reproductive Vitality · Empower Informed Healing

Use this checklist to explore overlooked aspects of reproductive health. It is not meant to diagnose but to bring awareness to areas that may be impacting your fertility journey.

Hormonal Imbalances & Cycle Irregularities

- Irregular or missing periods

- Painful or extremely heavy cycles

- Symptoms of estrogen dominance (e.g., breast tenderness, bloating, mood swings)

- Symptoms of low progesterone (e.g., short luteal phase, spotting before period)

- Low libido or vaginal dryness

- Signs of androgen excess (e.g., acne, facial hair, scalp hair thinning)

Nervous System & Stress Responses

- High perceived stress levels or chronic anxiety

- Trouble sleeping or insomnia

- History of trauma or emotional dysregulation

- Frequent "fight, flight, or freeze" experiences

- Poor emotional boundaries or constant caregiving

burnout

Somatic & Energetic Blocks

- Disconnection from womb, pelvic, or sexual awareness

- History of sexual trauma, shame, or suppression

- Pelvic floor tightness or pain during intimacy

- Difficulty accessing pleasure, joy, or embodiment

- Feeling emotionally "numb" or energetically "stuck" in the lower chakras

Nutrient Deficiencies & Digestive Imbalances

- Low intake of zinc, magnesium, B12, iron, or folate

- History of restrictive dieting, weight fluctuations, or eating disorders

- Bloating, gas, or inconsistent bowel movements

- Poor absorption or gut inflammation (IBS, SIBO, leaky gut)

- Use of PPIs, antacids, or birth control pills for long periods

Environmental & Toxic Exposure

- Daily use of plastic containers, bottled water, or canned foods

- Use of conventional cosmetics, perfumes, or cleaning products

- Regular exposure to endocrine disruptors (BPA, phthalates, parabens)

- Past or current mold exposure, heavy metals, or pesticides

- Limited or no detoxification support (sweating, liver-cleansing foods, etc.)

Underlying Conditions & Unexplored Diagnoses

- History of PCOS, endometriosis, or fibroids

- Thyroid imbalances (hypo or hyperthyroidism, Hashimoto's)

- Autoimmune disorders or family history of them

- Blood sugar instability or insulin resistance

- Undiagnosed or untreated STIs, BV, or pelvic inflammation

Relationship, Sexual, & Emotional Health

- Intimacy feels performative or disconnected from emotional safety

- Relationship stress, unspoken resentment, or attachment wounding

- Shame or guilt associated with sexuality or reproductive identity

- Feeling pressure, fear, or grief around conception

- Lack of joy, creativity, or inner sense of "receiving"

Reflection Questions

- Which of these areas surprised you the most?

- What are 2–3 items that feel most important to explore further?

- Where might you need support (e.g., practitioner, testing, therapy, rest)?

Fertility Assessment Checklist for Providers & Coaches

Root-Cause Insight · Functional Review · Whole-Person Approach

1. Menstrual Cycle Health

- Regular cycle (21–35 days)

- History of amenorrhea, dysmenorrhea, or irregular cycles

- PMS symptoms (cramping, mood changes, breast tenderness)

- Signs of anovulatory cycles (no mid-cycle temperature shift, short luteal phase)

- Use of hormonal contraceptives (past/present, duration)

- Recent discontinuation of hormonal birth control (within last 12 months)

2. Hormonal & Endocrine Function

- Signs of estrogen dominance (heavy bleeding, clots, fibroids, mood swings)

- Signs of progesterone deficiency (short luteal phase, spotting, anxiety, insomnia)

- Symptoms of androgen excess (facial hair, cystic acne, hair thinning)

- History of thyroid issues (cold intolerance, fatigue, irregular cycles)

- Insulin resistance or blood sugar instability

- Morning cortisol pattern (flat, elevated, reversed)

3. Nutritional & Digestive Health

- Nutrient-dense, whole foods-based diet

- Restrictive eating patterns or chronic dieting

- Digestive symptoms (bloating, gas, constipation, diarrhea)

- History of gut infections (candida, SIBO, parasites)

- Food sensitivities or intolerances (gluten, dairy, soy)

- Known micronutrient deficiencies (iron, B12, folate, zinc, magnesium)

4. Emotional Health & Stress Profile

- High stress lifestyle or Type A personality

- Unresolved trauma or PTSD

- Grief, loss, or history of miscarriage

- Emotional regulation challenges (irritability, overwhelm, avoidance)

- Current support system (partner, community, therapy)

- Mind-body tools currently in use (breathwork, meditation, journaling)

5. Somatic, Sexual & Pelvic Health

- Pelvic pain, tightness, or numbness

- History of sexual trauma or pain with intercourse

- Disconnection from body, sensuality, or reproductive organs

- Difficulty achieving arousal or orgasm

- Pelvic floor assessment completed (yes/no)

- Embodiment practices or movement (dance, yoga, somatic therapy)

6. Medical & Structural History

- Diagnosed conditions: PCOS, endometriosis, fibroids, adenomyosis

- Past surgeries (C-section, laparoscopies, D&C)

- Infections or untreated STIs

- Uterine abnormalities (septate uterus, tilted uterus, etc.)

- Genetic concerns or chromosomal issues

- Male partner fertility concerns (sperm analysis results)

7. Environmental & Lifestyle Exposures

- Use of non-toxic personal care & cleaning products

- Filtered water, glass containers, and minimal plastic use

- EMF exposure (phones on body, near Wi-Fi routers, etc.)

- Known exposure to mold, pesticides, or heavy metals

- Detox capacity supported (liver health, regular elimination, sweating)

- Alcohol, tobacco, or recreational drug use

8. Energetic & Spiritual Factors

- History of energetic or ancestral womb imprints

- Spiritual beliefs around conception and pregnancy

- Fear, guilt, or shame associated with motherhood or fertility

- Cord-cutting or ancestral healing practices used

- Chakra imbalances—especially root, sacral, and solar plexus

- Alignment with partner or inner divine masculine/ feminine

Provider Notes Section

- What stands out as the primary area for exploration?

- Which domains are most dysregulated?

- What testing, referrals, or lifestyle shifts are warranted?

- Are there cultural or spiritual considerations to honor in this client's path?

Male Hypofunction Laboratory Assessment Chart For Practitioners & Coaches

Lab Marker	Optimal Range	Clinical Relevance	Possible Imbalance Indications
Total Testosterone	600–900 ng/dL	Primary male androgen; critical for libido, mood, muscle mass, energy	<400 may indicate hypogonadism; fatigue, low libido, ED
Free Testosterone	15–25 ng/dL (or 2–3% of total)	Biologically active form; unbound and usable	Low free T with normal total T may suggest SHBG imbalance
Sex Hormone Binding Globulin (SHBG)	20–50 nmol/L	Binds testosterone; regulates free hormone	High SHBG = low free T; often elevated with aging, hyperthyroid
Luteinizing Hormone (LH)	2–9 IU/L	Stimulates testosterone production in testes	Low LH with low T = secondary hypogonadism; High LH = primary
Follicle-Stimulating Hormone (FSH)	1.5–12.4 IU/L	Spermatogenesis; Sertoli cell function	Elevated in testicular failure; low in pituitary dysfunction
Estradiol (E2, Sensitive Male Panel)	10–40 pg/mL	Estrogen balance; too low = bone/joint issues, too high = T suppression	Elevated with adiposity or aromatase excess
DHEA-Sulfate (DHEA-S)	250–600 mcg/dL (men <50)	Adrenal androgen precursor; vitality, libido, mood	Low = adrenal fatigue, aging; High = insulin resistance
Prolactin	<15 ng/mL	Inhibits gonadotropin release; linked to libido and mood	Elevated may suppress T production; check for pituitary issues
Cortisol (AM Serum)	6–18 µg/dL	Stress hormone impacting testosterone & DHEA	High cortisol can suppress gonadotropins & T production
Insulin (Fasting)	<8 uIU/mL	Insulin resistance affects SHBG, DHEA, estrogen	High insulin reduces SHBG, increases E2
Vitamin D (25-OH D)	50–80 ng/mL	Cofactor for testosterone synthesis & receptor function	Deficiency linked to low testosterone and fatigue
Zinc (Plasma/Serum)	70–120 µg/dL	Cofactor in testosterone synthesis and sperm production	Low levels impair fertility and hormone regulation

Optional Add-Ons for Functional Insight

Test	Purpose
Sperm Analysis	Volume, motility, morphology,

	count
Thyroid Panel (TSH, Free T3, Free T4, rT3)	Thyroid dysfunction often mimics low T symptoms
GI MAP or Stool Panel	Gut-liver axis assessment; estrogen reabsorption via beta-glucuronidase
Organic Acids Test (OAT)	Mitochondrial, neurotransmitter & nutrient cofactors relevant to testosterone and libido
Genetic Testing (e.g., SHBG SNPs, MTHFR, COMT)	Polymorphisms affecting hormone metabolism & clearance

Notes for Clinicians & Coaches

- Always **correlate labs with symptoms** (libido, vitality, mood, strength, cognitive performance).

- Run **AM blood draws** (7–10am) for hormone accuracy.

- Consider **salivary or DUTCH testing** for circadian rhythm, cortisol, and bioavailable hormones.

- **Repeat testing every 3–6 months** when adjusting protocols or tracking interventions.

Appendix C: Worksheets

Compatibility Worksheet: Exploring Alignment in Relationships

For Couples, Coaches, and Conscious Communicators

Section 1: Core Values & Beliefs

Instructions: Individually write your answers, then compare and discuss.

Topic	Partner A's Response	Partner B's Response	Alignment Level (Low – Medium – High)
Life Purpose & Vision			
Spiritual/Religious Beliefs			
Family & Children			
Finances & Wealth Goals			
Health & Wellness Values			
Career Ambitions			

Section 2: Communication & Emotional Expression

- We can talk openly about our feelings.

- We respect each other's boundaries during conflict.

- I feel emotionally safe and seen in this relationship.

- We use repair tools after disagreements.

- We validate each other's needs even when we disagree.

Reflection Prompt:
What communication patterns strengthen your connection?
What patterns need healing?

Section 3: Intimacy & Sexual Connection

- We discuss our desires, fantasies, and boundaries.

- We feel energetically and emotionally connected during intimacy.

- Our libidos are compatible or consciously negotiated.

- There is mutual pleasure, exploration, and consent.

- We check in after sex to deepen emotional safety.

What turns you on emotionally?

What makes you feel most connected during sex?

Section 4: Lifestyle & Nervous System Alignment

Trait	Partner A	Partner B	Notes
Introvert/Extrovert			
Cleanliness/Order			
Risk Tolerance			
Time Management Style			
Social Needs (alone vs. together time)			

Nutrition/Health
Priorities

Stress Coping Styles

What nervous system state do you bring into the relationship most often—calm, anxious, shut down, reactive? How do you co-regulate?

Section 5: Energetic & Spiritual Alignment

- We honor each other's soul paths and healing journeys.

- We feel spiritually or cosmically connected.

- We engage in rituals, prayer, or energy practices together.

- We share similar views on the sacredness of love and sex.

- We understand our masculine/feminine dynamics and seek harmony.

Energetic Insight Prompt:
How does your partner affect your energy field—do they calm, energize, or dysregulate you?

Navigating Compatibility

- **Where are you most aligned?**
- **Where do you experience contrast or tension?**
- **Are your differences complementary or conflicting?**
- **What would deepen your compatibility right now—individually and as a couple?**

Partner Compatibility Worksheet Assessment

Name (Partner A): _____

Name (Partner B): _____

Date: _____

Instructions:

Each partner completes the worksheet independently first. Then, compare answers and discuss similarities, differences, and opportunities for growth. Use the rating scales and reflection prompts to guide your dialogue.

1. Emotional Compatibility

Question	Partner A	Partner B
I feel emotionally safe with my partner. (1–5)		
We know how to repair after conflict. (1–5)		
We are attuned to each other's moods and needs. (1–5)		
I feel supported when I am vulnerable. (1–5)		
We can express emotions without fear of judgment. (1–5)		

Reflection Prompt:
What emotional patterns have strengthened your bond? Which patterns need healing?

2. Sexual Compatibility

Question	Partner A	Partner B

Our libidos are aligned or consciously negotiated. (1–5)

We can express sexual needs without shame. (1–5)

There is mutual exploration, consent, and satisfaction. (1–5)

Our intimate moments feel emotionally connected. (1–5)

We understand and respect each other's boundaries and rhythms. (1–5)

Reflection Prompt:
What does satisfying intimacy look like for you, and how is it created or blocked?

3. Lifestyle Compatibility

Topic	Partner A's Response	Partner B's Response	Alignment (Low – High)
Daily routines			
Nutrition & health habits			
Financial values			
Home cleanliness			
Social life preferences			

Bonus Prompt:
How do your nervous systems feel around each other—safe, drained, or activated?

4. Spiritual & Energetic Compatibility

Question	Partner A	Partner B
We share or respect each other's spiritual beliefs. (1–5)		
We can engage in sacred rituals or practices together. (1–5)		
Our energy feels aligned or harmonious during deep connection. (1–5)		
We experience each other as soul companions. (1–5)		
We hold space for each other's healing journeys. (1–5)		

Reflection Prompt:
What does sacred intimacy mean to you? Do you feel you experience it together?

5. Future Vision & Shared Goals

Statement	Agree/Disagree	Notes
We share similar long-term goals and values.		
We have compatible views on children, parenting, or family structures.		
We have a mutual understanding of roles in career/home balance.		
We talk openly about finances, investments, and		

abundance mindsets.

We're on the same page about the type of life we're building together.

Final Assessment Summary

Where are we most aligned?

_____

_____

_____

Where are we experiencing contrast or growth edges?

_____

_____

_____

What practices can support our continued compatibility?

_____

_____

_____

Are we choosing each other from wholeness or fear of lack?

_____

_____

_____

Appendix D: Sample Protocols

Hormone Balance Daily Routine

- Morning: Ashwagandha (adaptogen), magnesium glycinate, hydration with lemon water
- Midday: 20-minute sun exposure, high-protein lunch, zinc and omega-3
- Evening: Gentle movement, guided meditation, dim lights, magnesium bath soak

PCOS Support Protocol

- Inositol supplement (2g/day)
- Chromium and NAC
- Anti-inflammatory diet (low glycemic, dairy-free)
- Weekly castor oil packs over ovaries

Male Hypogonadism Support

- Strength training 3x/week
- Tongkat Ali and Vitamin D3
- Mindfulness breathing practices for cortisol regulation
- Functional lab panel every 3–6 months

Detoxification Support

- Milk thistle, dandelion, burdock tea
- Dry brushing and lymphatic massage
- Infrared sauna or Epsom salt baths 3x/week
- Eliminate plastic containers, processed foods, and artificial fragrances

Principles of a Microbiome Reset

- **Prebiotic-Rich Foods**: garlic, leeks, onions, asparagus, green bananas, oats

- **Probiotic-Rich Foods**: fermented veggies, kefir, coconut yogurt, kimchi, sauerkraut

- **Polyphenols & Antioxidants**: berries, green tea, cacao, turmeric, olive oil

- **Diverse Plant Fibers**: variety of legumes, cruciferous veggies, leafy greens

- **Avoid**: refined sugar, processed food, seed oils, artificial sweeteners, alcohol

7-Day Meal Plan

Each day includes breakfast, lunch, dinner, and one gut-supportive snack or drink.

Day 1: Gut Awakening

Breakfast: Green Gut Smoothie

- Spinach, avocado, green apple, flaxseed, chia, kefir, ginger, lemon

Lunch: Lentil & Vegetable Stew

- Carrots, celery, garlic, turmeric, thyme, lentils, bone broth or veggie broth

Dinner: Grilled Salmon over Arugula Salad

- Arugula, red cabbage, cucumber, pumpkin seeds, olive oil, lemon

Snack: Sauerkraut + ¼ avocado on rice crackers

Day 2: Fiber & Ferment Focus

Breakfast: Overnight Oats

- Rolled oats, chia, coconut yogurt, blueberries, walnuts,

cinnamon

Lunch: Quinoa Power Bowl

- Quinoa, roasted sweet potato, broccoli, chickpeas, tahini dressing

Dinner: Miso Soup with Bok Choy and Seaweed

- Fermented miso, tofu, scallions, shiitake mushrooms, bok choy, seaweed

Snack: Cucumber slices with hummus and hemp seeds

Day 3: Anti-Inflammatory Reset

Breakfast: Chia Pudding

- Chia, unsweetened almond milk, raspberries, cacao nibs, cinnamon

Lunch: Mediterranean Wrap

- Collard green wrap with hummus, grilled veggies, olives, sprouts

Dinner: Turmeric-Spiced Cauliflower & Lentil Curry

- Cauliflower, turmeric, ginger, garlic, lentils, coconut milk

Snack: Kombucha or coconut kefir + handful of almonds

Day 4: Root & Repair

Breakfast: Sweet Potato Hash

- Sweet potato, onions, kale, eggs (or tempeh), rosemary

Lunch: Cabbage & Apple Slaw with Wild-Caught Sardines

- Green & purple cabbage, green apple, carrots, lemon, olive oil

Dinner: Herb-Roasted Chicken with Garlic Brussels Sprouts

- Bone-in chicken thighs, rosemary, garlic, olive oil, roasted sprouts

Snack: Pear slices + sunflower seed butter

Day 5: Diverse Digestion

Breakfast: Plant-Based Green Smoothie

- Swiss chard, pear, kiwi, avocado, ground flax, mint, spirulina

Lunch: Lentil Tacos in Lettuce Cups

- Spiced lentils, avocado, salsa, red onion, cilantro

Dinner: Grilled Tempeh Stir Fry

- Tempeh, snow peas, carrots, scallions, coconut aminos, sesame oil

Snack: Kimchi + roasted seaweed snacks

Day 6: Microbial Diversity Day

Breakfast: Mango Coconut Chia Bowl

- Chia, coconut milk, mango, pumpkin seeds, lime zest

Lunch: Hearty Veggie & Bean Chili

- Kidney beans, black beans, peppers, onions, zucchini, cumin

Dinner: Roasted Beets & Citrus Salad + Seared Trout

- Roasted beets, orange slices, arugula, pistachios, goat cheese

Snack: Pickled veggies + digestive herbal tea (e.g., fennel, ginger, mint)

Day 7: Integration & Intuition

Breakfast: Yogurt Parfait

- Unsweetened coconut or almond yogurt, berries, flaxseed, cacao nibs

Lunch: Wild Rice & Mushroom Bowl

- Wild rice, sautéed mushrooms, kale, onions, garlic, miso-tahini drizzle

Dinner: Stuffed Acorn Squash

- Acorn squash filled with quinoa, cranberries, kale, pecans, herbs

Snack: Golden milk (turmeric, ginger, cinnamon, black pepper, almond milk)

Hydration & Lifestyle Tips

- Start each day with warm lemon water

- Drink herbal teas that support digestion (peppermint, dandelion, licorice)

- 1 tbsp apple cider vinegar in water before heavy meals (if tolerated)

- Avoid distractions while eating (no phones/screens)

- Walk 10–20 mins after meals to support motility

Fertility Recovery Plan

"Reclaim your womb. Reclaim your rhythm. Reclaim your right to create."

1. Nervous System Regulation & Stress Recovery

Unresolved chronic stress directly impacts ovulation, hormone production, and sperm quality. Restoring nervous system balance is a foundational step in fertility recovery.

Tools & Techniques:

- **Daily NSI Practice**: Vagal toning, breathwork, or cold exposure

- **Cortisol Management**: Adaptogens (ashwagandha, holy basil), magnesium glycinate

- **Sleep Hygiene**: 7–9 hrs, screen-free 90 min before bed, herbal teas (chamomile, lemon balm)

- **Somatic Therapy**: TRE, EMDR, or somatic experiencing to clear trauma stored in the body

Try: 10-min guided yoga nidra to reset the HPA axis

2. Nutritional & Functional Medicine Support

Food is not just fuel—it's information for hormonal harmony. A whole food fertility-supportive diet addresses nutrient deficiencies, insulin resistance, and inflammation.

Key Components:

- **Anti-Inflammatory Diet**: Eliminate seed oils, sugar, dairy (if inflammatory), gluten (if sensitive)

- **Increase**: Leafy greens, root vegetables, omega-3s (flax, walnuts, wild fish), bone broth

- **Fertility Nutrients**:

  - Zinc, Vitamin D, Selenium, B6, B12, Folate (Methylated)

  - Iron, Magnesium, Choline, Iodine

Herbal Allies:

- **Chasteberry (Vitex)**: Normalizes LH and progesterone in luteal phase

- **Maca Root**: Adaptogenic, hormone-balancing, libido-enhancing

- **Red Raspberry Leaf**: Uterine toning

- **Nettles**: Mineral-rich, especially iron

3. Functional Testing (Optional but Insightful)

Work with a fertility-informed provider to test:

Test	What It Reveals
DUTCH Hormone Test	Estrogen, progesterone, cortisol, DHEA balance
AMH	Ovarian reserve
Thyroid Panel	TSH, Free T3, Free T4, Reverse T3, antibodies

Vitamin D, Iron/ Ferritin	Nutrient levels
GI Map or GI Effects	Gut inflammation, infections, leaky gut
Sperm Analysis	Count, motility, morphology

4. Cycle Awareness & Ovulation Tracking

Knowing your body's rhythms is an act of sovereignty.

Track:

- **Basal Body Temperature (BBT)**

- **Cervical Mucus**: Egg-white mucus indicates fertility

- **Luteinizing Hormone (LH) Surge**: Use OPKs

- **Cycle Phases**:

    o   Follicular (Day 1–13) – Build

    o   Ovulatory (Day 14–16) – Peak fertility

    o   Luteal (Day 17–28) – Rest & reflect

Use a fertility journal or apps like Kindara, Tempdrop, or Clue

5. Emotional & Relationship Healing

Fertility struggles often impact self-worth, intimacy, and connection.

Explore:

- **Womb Healing Ceremonies or Steam Rituals**

- **Therapeutic Journaling**: Write letters to your womb or future child

- **Couples Communication Practices**: NVC (Nonviolent Communication), vulnerability dialogues

- **Grief Work**: Honor pregnancy loss, fertility trauma, or unmet expectations

"Your womb remembers. Your womb heals."

6. Environmental Detox

Endocrine disruptors in everyday items can sabotage fertility.

Reduce Exposure To:

- **Plastics (BPA, phthalates)**: Use glass/stainless steel

- **Pesticides**: Eat organic when possible (Dirty Dozen)

- **Toxins in beauty/cleaning products**: Switch to non-toxic, EWG-verified brands

- **EMFs**: Limit laptops on lap, turn off Wi-Fi at night

7. Energetic & Spiritual Reconnection

Your womb is not just anatomical—it's energetic.

Practices:

- **Womb Meditation**: Visualize golden healing light entering your womb space

- **Yoni Steaming**: With herbs like mugwort, lavender, calendula, basil (cycle-specific)

- **Affirmations**:

  o   "I trust my body's divine timing."

  o   "My womb is wise, vibrant, and receptive."

  o   "I release shame and welcome sacred creation."

Align with lunar cycles for menstruation and ovulation rituals

Functional Supplement Toolkit

"Support the body's innate intelligence with precision, purpose, and plant-powered potency."

⚠ **Disclaimer:** This list is for educational purposes only. Dosages and use should be customized by a qualified practitioner based on labs, symptoms, and medical history.

1. Hormone Harmony & Cycle Regulation

Supplement	Typical Dosage	Benefits
Chaste Tree (Vitex agnus-castus)	200–400 mg daily (AM)	Regulates luteal phase, supports progesterone, helpful for PMS and cycle irregularities.
DIM (Diindolylmethane)	100–200 mg daily	Supports estrogen metabolism and detoxification via liver pathways.
Evening Primrose Oil	1,000–1,500 mg daily	Supports cervical fluid, inflammation, and hormone balance in the luteal phase.
Calcium D-Glucarate	250–500 mg daily	Promotes estrogen clearance through the glucuronidation pathway.
Omega-3 (EPA/DHA)	1,000–2,000 mg daily	Anti-inflammatory, hormone balancing, supports cervical mucus and egg quality.

2. Libido & Sexual Energy Boosters

Supplement	Typical Dosage	Benefits

Maca Root (Lepidium meyenii)	500–1,000 mg 1–2x/day	Enhances libido, stamina, adrenal support, mood balance.
Ashwagandha (Withania somnifera)	300–600 mg 1–2x/day	Adaptogen that reduces cortisol and improves testosterone/libido.
Tribulus terrestris	250–500 mg daily	May boost libido and ovarian stimulation; shown helpful in both genders.
Horny Goat Weed (Epimedium)	250–500 mg daily	Natural PDE5 inhibitor that enhances blood flow and libido.
L-Arginine	2–3g before intimacy or daily	Improves nitric oxide, blood flow, and arousal.

3. Fertility & Reproductive Support

Supplement	Typical Dosage	Benefits
CoQ10 (Ubiquinol form)	100–300 mg daily	Supports egg/sperm quality and mitochondrial energy.
Myoinositol + D-Chiro Inositol	2,000–4,000 mg/day	Improves ovulation, insulin sensitivity, and egg quality (esp. PCOS).
N-Acetyl Cysteine (NAC)	600–1,200 mg/day	Supports cervical mucus, detox, and egg health.
Prenatal with Methylfolate	As directed (1–2 caps/day)	Foundational multivitamin with active B vitamins, iron, iodine, zinc.
L-Carnitine	1,000–2,000 mg/day	Enhances sperm motility and female fertility by boosting mitochondrial

function.

4. Nervous System & Stress Regulation

Supplement	Typical Dosage	Benefits
Magnesium Glycinate or L-Threonate	200–400 mg at night	Calms nervous system, improves sleep, hormone and cortisol regulation.
L-Theanine	100–200 mg 1–2x/day	Promotes alpha brain waves, calm focus, reduces anxiety.
Rhodiola Rosea	200–400 mg AM	Adaptogen for stress resilience and mental performance.
Phosphatidylserine	100–200 mg at night	Blunts evening cortisol, improves sleep and memory.
GABA (PharmaGABA or liposomal)	100–300 mg as needed	Supports parasympathetic activation, relaxation, and calm.

5. Functional Mushrooms & Immune Balance

Supplement	Typical Dosage	Benefits
Reishi	500–1,000 mg PM	Adrenal support, immune regulation, deep sleep.
Cordyceps	500–1,000 mg AM	Boosts stamina, energy, oxygenation, libido.
Lion's Mane	500–1,000 mg daily	Supports neuroplasticity, cognition, and emotional regulation.

Appendix E: Libido & Hormone Tracking Tools

"When we track our inner rhythms, we reclaim our power to heal, harmonize, and honor our body's truth."

Daily/Weekly Tracker Template

Date	Menstrual Cycle Day	Libido Level (0–10)	Mood/ Emotions	Energy Level (Low/Mid/ High)	Cervical Mucus	Sleep Quality	Notes (Stressors, Intimacy, Self-care)

Libido Observation Prompts

Each day or week, use these questions for deeper reflection:

1. **How would you describe your desire today?**

   o None, Low, Curious, Warm, Strong, Overflowing

2. **Did you feel emotionally connected to your body and/or partner?**

   o Yes / No / Somewhat

3. **What sensual or erotic thoughts, dreams, or feelings arose?**

---

4. **What nervous system state do you feel you were in most of the day?**

   o Fight / Flight / Freeze / Rest / Pleasure

5. **Was there any guilt, shame, or resistance toward your arousal?**

   o If yes, journal why.

Hormone & Cycle Symptom Log

Hormonal Symptom	Severity (0–10)	Notes
Breast tenderness		
PMS/PMDD		
Mid-cycle cramps		
Headaches/Migraines		
Vaginal dryness		
Mood swings		
Bloating		
Acne or skin flare-ups		
Sleep disruption		
Digestive changes		

4-Phase Cycle Energy & Libido Patterns

Use this to track trends across your menstrual cycle:

Phase	Approx. Days	Typical Libido	Energy	Emotional Themes
Menstrual	1–5	Low / inward	Low	Release, reflection
Follicular	6–13	Building	Moderate	Hope, motivation
Ovulatory	14–16	Peak	High	Radiance, confidence
Luteal	17–28	Fluctuating	Decreasing	Sensitivity, truth

Optional Hormone Testing Log

Test	Date	Result	Notes
Estradiol (E2)			
Progesterone			
Testosterone			
DHEA			
Cortisol (AM/PM)			
Thyroid Panel			
Vitamin D			

Integration & Reflection Journal Prompts

- What patterns are emerging in my libido across different cycle phases?

- What activities help me feel turned on, empowered, or embodied?

- Are there emotional wounds (shame, fear, rejection) that influence my libido?

- How does my relationship with pleasure reflect my relationship with power?

- What is my body asking for today?

Appendix F: Healing Roadmap: Reclaiming Hormonal Balance, Connection, and Wholeness

This roadmap is a synthesis of the practices, tools, and insights explored throughout the book. It serves as a step-by-step integrative guide for anyone looking to reclaim their hormonal health, deepen intimacy, and live in alignment with their true essence.

Step 1: Awareness & Assessment

- Begin with functional testing (hormones, nutrients, thyroid, inflammation markers)
- Complete libido and cycle tracking logs
- Identify energetic imbalances (excess masculine/feminine)

Step 2: Nervous System Regulation

- Breathwork (box breathing, 4-7-8 method)
- Somatic grounding practices (EFT, TRE, body scanning)
- Digital detox to reduce cortisol load

Step 3: Functional Nutrition & Detox

- Transition to whole foods anti-inflammatory diet
- Use adaptogens and herbal supports tailored to hormonal needs (e.g., ashwagandha, chasteberry)
- Support liver detoxification: cruciferous vegetables, water intake, magnesium

Step 4: Somatic & Sexual Reconnection

- Explore solo somatic practices: mirror work, mindful touch
- Engage in sacred sexual rituals with partners
- Reframe pleasure as healing, not performance

Step 5: Relationship Rebalancing

- Practice emotional availability and nonviolent communication
- Address sexual compatibility and attachment dynamics
- Create sacred space for intimacy and energy attunement

Step 6: Energetic Integration

- Journal daily: "Which part of me needs more love today?"
- Use chakra alignment meditations or sound healing
- Explore creative expression (dance, art, poetry) as energetic balancing tools

Step 7: Maintenance & Mastery

- Periodic re-testing and tracking symptoms
- Seasonal cleansing or spiritual renewal rituals
- Ongoing learning and evolving your embodiment journey

Suggested Weekly Healing Structure

Day	Focus Area	Practice Example
Monday	Nervous System	Guided breathwork + digital fasting
Tuesday	Nutrition & Gut Health	Anti-inflammatory meal prep + herbal tonic
Wednesday	Movement & Hormones	Qigong or strength training
Thursday	Emotional Intimacy	Journaling + inner child work

Friday	Sacred Sexuality	Solo or partnered sensuality exploration
Saturday	Creative Integration	Dance, painting, singing, writing
Sunday	Spiritual Connection	Meditation + energetic alignment practice

This roadmap is not a checklist—it is a compass. Let it guide you back to your body, your breath, and your truth.

10 Signs Your Hormones Are Under Attack (And What to Do About It)

By Dr. Deilen Michelle Villegas, Ph.D., DNM, HHP

Hormones don't just regulate your reproductive system —they're the biochemical messengers responsible for everything from mood and metabolism to libido, sleep, energy, and immunity. When they're under attack, the body speaks in symptoms. The question is: Are you listening?

1. Fatigue That Doesn't Go Away

Why: Cortisol dysregulation, adrenal fatigue, thyroid imbalance
What to Do:

- Prioritize deep rest and circadian-aligned sleep

- Support adrenals with B5, ashwagandha, vitamin C

- Remove caffeine dependence and consider salivary cortisol testing

2. Weight Gain (Especially Around the Belly)

Why: Insulin resistance, estrogen dominance, cortisol excess
What to Do:

- Follow a low-glycemic, anti-inflammatory diet

- Incorporate resistance training and intermittent fasting

- Add magnesium, berberine, and chromium support

3. Brain Fog & Forgetfulness

Why: Low progesterone, thyroid dysfunction, high

inflammation
What to Do:

- Optimize omega-3s and vitamin D

- Consider neuro-supportive herbs (ginkgo, lion's mane)

- Test T3, T4, and reverse T3—not just TSH

4. Mood Swings, Anxiety, or Depression

Why: Estrogen/progesterone imbalance, low testosterone, cortisol imbalances
What to Do:

- Practice somatic regulation (breathwork, TRE, vagal toning)

- Support GABA production with magnesium, B6, and taurine

- Balance blood sugar and increase protein intake

5. Low Libido

Why: Declining testosterone, stress, low DHEA or thyroid issues
What to Do:

- Use adaptogens like maca or tribulus

- Reignite desire through sacred sexuality & energetic intimacy

- Support with zinc, vitamin D, and nervous system repair

6. Irregular Periods or Menstrual Distress

Why: Estrogen dominance, progesterone deficiency, PCOS, perimenopause

What to Do:

- Track cycles using apps or journals

- Support liver detox with DIM, milk thistle, cruciferous veggies

- Seed cycle and explore yoni steaming protocols

7. Acne, Hair Loss, or Facial Hair

Why: Androgen excess, PCOS, insulin resistance
What to Do:

- Stabilize insulin with diet and inositol

- Balance androgens with spearmint tea, saw palmetto

- Check for gut dysbiosis or liver sluggishness

8. Digestive Issues

Why: Estrogen and cortisol impact gut permeability & microbiome
What to Do:

- Incorporate fermented foods, fiber, and digestive bitters

- Consider stool testing or SIBO assessment

- Lower stress and support the gut-brain axis

9. Trouble Sleeping

Why: Cortisol curve imbalances, melatonin suppression, perimenopause
What to Do:

- Create a hormone-supportive nighttime routine

- Use passionflower, glycine, or magnesium glycinate

- Limit screens and regulate blood sugar before bed

10. Infertility or Miscarriage History

Why: Progesterone deficiency, thyroid imbalance, high stress
What to Do:

- Do a full hormone and thyroid panel + micronutrient test

- Support uterine lining with vitamin E, omega-3s, and acupuncture

- Detox gently and consider fertility-specific herbal protocols

Toolkit Tip:

If you checked off 3 or more signs, your hormones are waving a red flag—not just whispering. It's time to support your body through nervous system repair, functional nutrition, hormone testing, and lifestyle recalibration.

DEILEN MICHELLE VILLEGAS, PH.D.

10 Holistic Tools for Erectile Vitality

Reclaiming Masculine Health, Pleasure & Power

By Dr. Deilen Michelle Villegas, Ph.D., DNM, HHP

Whether you're navigating age-related shifts, post-traumatic stress, chronic stress, or simply seeking to revitalize your vitality, erectile health is more than just circulation—it's nervous system regulation, hormone balance, blood flow, mental clarity, emotional connection, and spiritual embodiment. These tools support the *root, heart, and mind* of your vitality.

1. Pelvic Floor Therapy & Breathwork

Supports: Blood flow, muscle tone, and nerve signaling

- Practice **diaphragmatic breathing** with pelvic contractions (reverse Kegels included)

- Improve sacral nerve function and perineal circulation

2. Tongkat Ali & Ashwagandha Protocol

Supports: Testosterone, libido, and cortisol balance

- **Tongkat Ali:** 200–400 mg/day (cycling recommended)

- **Ashwagandha:** 600 mg/day reduces cortisol, improves sperm motility

Synergistic Effect: Enhances nitric oxide release and hormone production when paired with exercise

3. Red Light Therapy (Near-Infrared)

Supports: Mitochondrial function and blood vessel dilation

- Target perineal area for 10–15 minutes, 2–3x/week

- Improves ATP, testosterone synthesis, and penile vascular health

4. Mindful Arousal Training & Edging

Supports: Neurological mapping and stamina

- Delay climax through slow breathing and pause techniques

- Strengthens body-mind connection to reduce performance anxiety

5. Acupuncture & Auricular Therapy

Supports: Energy meridians, stress, and blood circulation

- Points: Kidney meridian, Ren 4, Ren 6, Liver 3

- Increases parasympathetic tone and improves erectile function over time

6. L-Arginine + Citrulline Combo

Supports: Nitric oxide (NO) production and vasodilation

- **L-Arginine:** 3,000–6,000 mg/day

- **L-Citrulline:** 1,000–2,000 mg/day
  Evidence: Combines well with pycnogenol for clinically supported erectile function improvement

7. Emotional Release Therapy (Somatic/Trauma-Informed)

Supports: Nervous system safety and performance pressure

- Techniques: TRE, somatic experiencing, inner child work

- Explore stored sexual shame or relational trauma stored in the pelvis

8. Sacred Sexuality & Presence Practices

Supports: Connection, pleasure without performance, and spiritual embodiment

- Eye gazing, heart-to-heart touch, and presence-centered lovemaking

- Activates oxytocin, relaxes sympathetic dominance, increases connection-based arousal

9. Microcirculation & Vascular Tonics

Supports: Blood vessel integrity and elasticity

- Herbal options: **Ginkgo biloba, cayenne, horse chestnut, hawthorn**

- Supports capillary tone and penile tissue oxygenation

10. Sleep & Testosterone Sync

Supports: Hormone production and adrenal repair

- Deep sleep (7–9 hrs) is critical for daily testosterone spikes

- Supplement: **Magnesium glycinate, GABA, or L-theanine** to support circadian balance

Daily Hormone & Libido Health Tracker

Track your biofeedback for 30 days to uncover your patterns, improve vitality, and build deeper body literacy.

Metric	Description	1–5 Scale / Notes
Morning Erection (YES/NO)	Was spontaneous arousal present upon waking?	☐ Yes ☐ No
Libido Level	Desire for intimacy (self or partnered)	①②③④⑤
Energy Level	Overall vitality, motivation, and drive	①②③④⑤
Sleep Quality	Depth and restfulness of sleep	①②③④⑤
Stress Level	Perceived emotional or physical stress	①②③④⑤
Mood	Emotional state upon waking and throughout day	✳☐☐☐☐ (select or describe)
Intimacy Experience (Optional)	Engaged in self or partnered intimacy?	☐ Yes ☐ No
Connection Quality	Emotional closeness or presence with partner	①②③④⑤
Physical Activity	What movement or exercise did you do today?	_____
Supplements Taken	List or check any key functional supplements	_____
Food Triggers or Wins	Note energy dips, libido shifts, or vitality after meals	_____
Hydration	Approx. how much water consumed?	_____ oz / liters
Reflection	How did your body feel	_____

today? Any insights?

Mood & Libido Key Scale (For Journalers)

Scale	Description
1	Very low, disconnected, fatigued
2	Mild desire but low arousal
3	Baseline, stable but neutral
4	Energized, present, mild spontaneous arousal
5	High desire, vitality, playful or romantic state

30-Day Progress Snapshot

At the end of the 30 days, reflect on:

- Which days had highest libido and energy?

- What foods or supplements preceded strong libido/ mood?

- What stressors or emotional triggers led to dips?

- What intimacy practices increased connection?

www.ingramcontent.com/pod-product-compliance
Lightning Source LLC
Chambersburg PA
CBHW071728270326
41928CB00013B/2600